The Healthcare CEO

And
Physician Burnout Syndrome

Amr Al-Hariri, MD

ISBN: **1517798825**
ISBN-13: **978-1517798826**

DEDICATION

To all the parents who are doing their best to maximize the potentials of their children…We, the parents, understand what you are trying to do.

CONTENTS

AMR AL-HARIRI, MD

I Invest in Positive, Let it Flow into Your Life

A practicing Neurologist in California with the following certifications:

American Board of Psychiatry and Neurology

American Board of Internal Medicine

American Board of Pediatrics

This book is the first in a series about improving outcomes in medicine. This is not a simple formula that can be followed, it is a continuous implementation process of positive attributes.

What do you call the situation of a physician that accept insurance or Medicare, employed or an independent contractor, and feels that reimbursement continues to decline unfairly, while unable to take action to change the situation?

I call it a "job misfit", this is the seed that carries the risk of evolving into a burn out syndrome.

This comprehensive book is a must investment in the career of physicians, and their families; it is likely to pay dividends for years to come in a much better quality of life and productivity.

This is a must read for physicians' spouses and partners. You may have thought you knew the physician you sleep next to very well. But we assure you, you did not!

If you are a CEO or executive, health care consultant, a manager in a health care facility or organization, a health insurance strategist, or a politician; and you have the gut feeling that the tools available for you to thrive are not working out... I can help you serve your clients (the patients) to the level that your conscious dictate. The first step is to understand the problem. This is what this book is about

Once you have the problem dissected it is your nature and skill to develop your own, situation unique, strategies to maximize your return on investment in your most valuable assets: The Physicians; not the hospital building or the state of the art MRI.

"The Healthcare CEO" series addresses your needs

You are sophisticated, educated, capable and dedicated; this is why you are the CEO, the manager, the executive or consultant.

This is why this series is so different, but the right one for you.

I present you with a collection of building blocks; each of them is a unique concept by itself. Each one of them can be plugged into your organization independently and make a difference. Yet you can build an amazing structure from the ground up using all these building blocks.

It is you, the CEO, the chief engineer of your company's culture structure that can decide which blocks, when, and how.

Physician Burnout Syndrome

1 WHAT IS BURNOUT SYNDROME

"Burnout," at its core is varying degrees of stress-induced unhappiness.

It is a psychological term indicating long-term exhaustion and diminished interest in work. Most experts connect it to chronic stress which is not being coped with well, but there is growing evidence that it is a multi-factorial syndrome.

Even though it is a widespread problem costing billions of dollars, burnout is not recognized as a distinct disorder in the DSM-5 due to the fact that it is problematically close to depressive disorders.

If you are a physician accepting insurance or Medicare and you feel that reimbursement continues to decline unfairly, and you are unable to take action to change the situation, then you should call that situation a "job misfit", and realize that as a result you are at risk for developing burn out syndrome.

This book is written with physicians in mind, as well as many of the health care professionals and workers who are at risk for Burn-

Out Syndrome, all of whom have their own unique variables and statistics. This book may be an excellent resource for them. The health care careers which are at a higher risk for burn-out are:

- Health Care CEOs
- Hospital administrators and executives
- Clinic and outpatient facility managers
- Medical students
- Emergency response personnel
- Dentists
- Nurses
- Social workers
- Mental health workers
- Psychologists
- Occupational therapists
- Speech therapists

You may want to start this book by reading this very helpful introduction to burnout syndrome, recommended from a reliable entity, *The American College of Surgeons Board of Governors' (B/G) Committee on Physician Competency and Health report.* They published this report in the *ACS* Bulletin in 2013, recommending that surgeons consider the following self-assessment statements to determine if surgeon is vulnerable to burnout:

- I find meaning in my work

- I protect time away from work with my spouse, family, and friends

- I focus on what is most important to me in life

- I try to take a positive outlook on things

- I take vacations

- I participate in recreation/hobbies/exercise

- I talk with family, significant other, or friends about how I am feeling

- I have developed an approach/philosophy to dealing with patients' suffering and death

- I seek to strike a balance between my personal and professional life

- I look forward to retirement

- I discuss stressful aspects of work with colleagues

- I nurture the religious/spiritual aspects of myself

- I am involved in non-patient care activities (for example, research, education, and administration)

- I engage in contemplative practices or other mindfulness activities, such as meditation or narrative medicine

- I engage in reflective writing or other journaling technique

The more positive the responses, the less likely surgeons are to suffer from burnout, depression, suicidal ideation, decreased professional and personal quality of life, and abuse of alcohol or other drugs.

Hopefully by now you are intrigued and are considering investing in this self-help book. It is not your typical self-help book that has been filled with "fluff" in order to fatten the chapters and make it look worth the price tag.

It is not a book filled with clichés and a few banal pointers that promise to change your life.

Rather, this is a book written with your high IQ in mind; for the most part it presents you with dilemmas that are intended to trigger your brain into more directed self-reflection and soul searching.

Burnout is a very well known, well researched syndrome in the corporate world, but it is a relative newcomer in the physician's world. The most recent article on the subject was published in "Neurology" 2014 and it brushed on burn out syndrome among neurologists. There have been many articles over the past ten years that addressed this subject, but our best estimates indicate that burn out syndrome did not become a real issue for physicians as a group until the early 1990s.

Physicians did not start to recognize burnout as a serious threat to the nation's health, and their profession collectively, until possibly the early 2000s. We speculate the reason for that is that more and more MDs started to pursue MBAs at that time. Through the MBA courses, they were exposed to the well-recognized "Burn out Syndrome" as it exists in the corporate world.
As the numbers of physicians pursuing MBA degrees increased, there was a realization, an awakening if you will, that the features of burnout syndrome held many similarities to the signs and symptoms afflicting the physicians' work force. Physicians started

to compare the impact of burnout on the corporate work force, to the impact on their own productivity, and self-satisfaction as a group.

To put it all in a different prospective, doctors may not have been ready to acknowledge this syndrome as a real epidemic infecting the physicians' community, if not for the accelerating pressures imposed on their profession by a rapidly changing, increasingly regulated health care environment. Also in play was the input of visionary physician colleagues who were seeking MBA degrees so that they could spearhead efforts to manage the health care crisis.

In my opinion, these efforts continue to be individualistic and self-directed in nature, and for the most part lack a collective impact. These unscientific conclusions on our part are based on the constant increase in numbers of physicians who identify themselves as afflicted by at least one of the three common criteria for the accurate recognition of burn out syndrome.

Furthermore, studies have suggested that burnout is more prevalent among physicians than the general population or other professions with similar years of education.

Nearly half of physicians struggle with burn out syndrome

The study published in Archives of Internal Medicine 2012 addressed the following subject:

Burnout and Satisfaction with Work-Life Balance Among US

Physicians Relative to the General US Population

Of the 27276 Physicians who received invitations to participate in the study, 7288 completed the surveys.

Of those 7288 physicians, researchers found that 45.8% reported experiencing at least one symptom of serious burnout, such as emotional exhaustion, depersonalization and a low sense of personal accomplishment. Of the surveyed physicians, the study compared 6,179 practicing doctors ages 29 to 65 with 3,442 workers of the same age group in other fields. Doctors had a higher risk of emotional exhaustion (32.1% versus 23.5%) and overall burnout (37.9% versus 27.8%).

The study also found significant differences in burnout by specialty. Some of the highest rates were among physicians serving on the "front lines" of medicine in family medicine, general internal medicine and emergency medicine.

Phases of Burn Out Syndrome in The Corporate World

Psychologists **Herbert Freudenberger** and Gail North have theorized that the burnout process can be divided into 12 phases, which are not necessarily followed sequentially.

These phases are:

1- The Compulsion to prove oneself
2- Working Harder

3- Neglecting One's Needs

4- Displacement of Conflicts

5- Revision of Values

6- Denial of Emerging Problems

7- Withdrawal

8- Obvious Behavioral Changes, noticed by everyone at work

9- Depersonalization and losing the feeling of value in themselves or others

10- Inner Emptiness that may result in indulging in other activities that can fill the void like overeating, sex, alcohol, or drugs.

11- Depression

12- Burnout Syndrome

Burnout in its full presentation is characterized by decreased mental energy, absenteeism, high turnover, and reduced job satisfaction.

Three elements constitute burnout:

(1) Emotional exhaustion

(2) Depersonalization

(3) Low personal accomplishment

I believe that there are different stages/degrees of this syndrome, and it becomes a quality of life issue for physicians much earlier than is described in the 3 elements of full blown burnout mentioned above. In our opinion the signal of this critical early stage is when a physician stops having fun practicing medicine.

Productivity is Different for Physicians, something CEOs rarely understand

In my opinion, "Productivity" for a physician is different from that of a general worker or professional. There are no scientific papers we know of to support our claims. However, the practice of medicine is an art, and each patient is their own unique project to the practicing physician. Physicians invest in this human project a portion of their knowledge, a portion of their emotions, a portion of their life experience, and a portion of their time.(If you were to write a short story about the patient, you might call it "Soap Note".) There is a significant human emotional investment, as well as a deep feeling of responsibility, deep in the physician's conscious.

On the other hand, when a financial advisor makes a decision to buy or sell stocks, or when a CEO makes a decision to hire, fire, or invest capital in a new hospital, the common factor among is lack of human emotional investment. Those decisions are all about the numbers and the bottom line.

Yes, sometimes there is significant consideration to human issues, but in our opinion this is completely different from the emotional investment we addressed earlier.

So I am going to define productivity differently and uniquely for physicians, and digress from the corporate definition. We are describing "human project productivity", rather than item productivity. Each project includes many different items.

Let us put this into prospective using an example of your daily practice.

Your daily schedule says you are supposed to see a patient every 15 minutes.

In my opinion the morning sheet should say:

You have a human project to complete every 15 minutes.

Can you tell the difference?

But actually this is not the right way to say it! Surprised? You should be.

The morning schedule should say:

You have a human project to complete every 15 minutes for the next 8 hours, at the very least. We will give you an hour to eat lunch, while you are still catching up on your notes. This will include some weekends and many nights.

You are expected not to make any mistakes, and expected at all times to honor your oath "do not harm". You will go back to your family after work and be a fantastic mom, wife, husband, dad, or partner. Oh, and by the way, you will do this for the next 40 years.

Whether or not you think this scenario is nonsense, it is actually the first tool in the physician self-help, self-healing process.

The above summary of a physician's career is one of the most important tools you should start to utilize. The tool is to simply remind oneself of how important a physician's job is on a day to day basis. Physicians are notorious for down playing what they do.

Can you as a physician retrain yourself, at least once a week, to say I have helped that many people this week?

No?

You cannot?

Not surprised at all.

Is this a very self-absorbing task for you?

This may sound like a very romantic way of approaching medical practice.

But finding value in the daily practice of medicine is one of the very important tools available to physicians in overcoming burnout.

We are going to address this subject in much more depth in other chapters of this book.

Consequences of Burn out Syndrome

Impact on the Physician's Quality of Life:

- Absenteeism
- Intention to give up practicing clinical medicine
- Quality of personal life declines
- Family relationships decline
- Alcohol abuse
- Drug abuse
- Extra-marital affairs
- The perception of having made medical mistakes
- Empathy
- Depression
- Anxiety
- Insomnia
- Early retirement

Impact on Patient Care and Physician Performance:

- The perception of having made medical mistakes
- Actually making more frequent medical mistakes
- Decreased productivity
- Increased utilization medical resources
- Devaluation of the patient-physician relationship to become a mechanical customer-provider relationship. This is a grey

area when it comes to burnout. We think that the aggressive attempts of managers to streamline patient-physician encounters in order to maximize their version of productivity and the bottom line, is a major factor in the erosion of the patient-physician relationship. In our opinion, this is one of the most important factors that contribute to burnout syndrome. We also believe that the devaluation of the patient-physician relationship is also a result of the declining reimbursement of Medicare and private insurers, and the RVU system which we believe has consistently failed to be fair to the cognitive medical specialties. This brings us back to our provocative statement at the beginning of the chapter:

"If you are a physician accepting insurance or Medicare and you feel that reimbursement continues to decline unfairly, and you are unable to take action to change the situation, then you should call that situation a "job misfit", and realize that as a result you are at risk for developing burn out syndrome."

2 EXPLORING THE BUIDLING BLOCKS

What is different about physicians that make them more prone to burnout than other professionals? When addressing this issue, it is best to compile building blocks of facts, and then draw conclusions based on these facts.

Building block #1

Specialties on the front line have higher rates of burnout, that is, internal medicine, family practice, and emergency medicine.

This was addressed in a paper published in Archives of Internal Medicine in 2012.

Archives of Internal Medicine. 2012 Oct 8; 172(18):1377-85.

Burnout and satisfaction with work-life balance among US physicians relative to the general US population.

Shanafelt TD1, Boone S, Tan L, Dyrbye LN, Sotile W, Satele D, West CP, Sloan J, Oreskovich MR.

In this study, the American Medical Association Physician Masterfile was used to invite 27,276 physicians to participate in a survey. 7,288 physicians (26.7%) completed their surveys. The

Maslach Burnout Inventory was used to assess burnout syndrome.

A- 45.8% of physicians reported at least 1 symptom of burnout.

B- Substantial differences in burnout were observed by specialty, with the highest rates among physicians at the front line of care access; family medicine, general internal medicine, and emergency medicine.

C- Compared with a probability-based sample of 3,442 working US adults, physicians were more likely to have symptoms of burnout (37.9% vs. 27.8%) and to be dissatisfied with work-life balance (40.2% vs. 23.2%).

D- The highest level of education completed also related to burnout in a pooled multivariate analysis adjusted for age, sex, relationship status, and hours worked per week. Compared with high school graduates, individuals with an MD or DO degree were at increased risk for burnout with an odds ratio of 1.36. For individuals with a bachelor's degree the odd ratio was 0.80, and for those with a master's degree the odd ratio was 0.71. Those with a professional or doctoral degree other than an MD or DO, had an odd ratio of 0.64, and were at lower risk for burnout.

Building Block #2

Burnout among neurologists is at a high of 50%, according to a paper published in "Neurology" in 2014. This rate is higher than other specialty groups, and is as high as the burnout rate found in the front-line specialties.

Neurology - Physician burnout A neurologic crisis

Bruce Sigsbee, MD and James L. Bernat, MD Correspondence to Dr. Sigsbee: bsigsbee@aan.com

Published November 5, 2014

What is also very interesting is the extensive efforts of the governing authorities in the specialty of neurology over the past few years, to convince Medicare to recognize neurology as a primary care specialty. This effort did not materializes in a vacuum. In other words, it was not just an effort on the part of neurologists to get the 10% higher compensation recently built into primary care specialties by Medicare. No, the concerted effort to be considered a primary care specialty comes from a genuine feeling that neurologists, who are cognitive specialists rather than procedure oriented specialists, are becoming the primary care providers for complex neurology patients. Neurology practice characteristics are becoming very much like a primary care practice characteristics. Regardless of this, these specialists are suffering from ongoing cuts in reimbursement for neurology procedures.

I speculate that the shift in practice that is moving Neurology closer to primary care is also moving the burnout rate among neurologists closer to that of their primary care colleagues. As such, they are experiencing burnout at a higher rate than their colleagues in other specialties.

Building Block #3

Decline in physician ownership.

This was brought on by the 1990s rush of hospitals to corner a market share of patients. In order to corner the market and build as large a patient volume as possible, hospitals started buying primary care practices, thereby transforming practice owner physicians into employee physicians.

This period of acquiring primary care practices lasted for a few years, before hospitals started shedding them. Hospitals had spent enormous capital on these acquisitions. Yet, they found that practice managers had difficulty maintaining productivity at previous levels. Practice operations had changed along with the physician's status from stockholder to employee. This resulted in a period of significant tension between physicians and hospital management.

This is the same period when HMOs began to grow rapidly. Utilization management burdens became a fact of life in the day-to-day practice of medicine.

History is once again repeating itself as hospitals rush to evolve into world class systems like the Mayo Clinic. At the root of this is the need of every hospital, and the parent institutions or systems, to prepare for market changes brought on by Obama Care. As a result, there is now tremendous growth in the existence of medical foundations that can legally hire physicians, using hospital money. This trend is transforming most new physicians' jobs, especially in urban areas, into employment positions in foundations or hospital affiliated large multi-specialty clinics. The consequence of this is that physicians have no ownership potential, further diminishing the share of physician ownership in healthcare assets.

Physician ownership of healthcare assets has been looked upon unfavorably by government and regulating agencies, as evidenced in the "Stark Law" legislation that was passed in the early 1990s.

Amazingly, right or wrong, a "business approach" has been adapted by both government and regulating agencies as they promote "stockholders and investors" rather than physicians, in owning the assets of health care.

Building Block #4

Decline in Physicians' real Income.

This is an ongoing reality and one that hits most primary care physicians. This too began in the 1990s. Between 1995 and 2003, the average physician net income from the practice of medicine declined about 7 percent after adjusting for inflation, according to

HSC's nationally representative 2004-05 Community Tracking Study Physician Survey.

Primary care physicians and surgeons fared the worst in keeping pace with inflation, while medical specialists fared the best. After adjusting for inflation, medical specialist' incomes have remained virtually unchanged since the mid-1990s. In contrast, primary care physicians—already the lowest earning of all physicians—have lost substantial ground (-10.2%) to inflation since the mid-1990s. Surgical specialists also experienced a significant reduction of more than 8 percent in real incomes between 1995 and 2003.

Negative real income trends for physicians stand in stark contrast to the trends experienced by workers in professional, specialty and technical occupations. Between 1995 and 2003, wages and salaries for these workers increased about 7 percent after adjusting for inflation. The divergence in income trends between physicians and other professional workers, which was especially striking in the 1995-1999 period, narrowed somewhat from 1999 to 2003, but physicians still lagged behind fellow professionals.

(Changes in wage/salary income for private sector "professional, specialty and technical" workers are based on the Bureau of Labor Statistics (BLS) Employment Cost Index (http://data.bls.gov/labjava/outside.jsp?survey=ec). Data were adjusted for inflation using the BLS online inflation calculator (http://146.142.4.24/cgi-bin/cpicalc.pl).

This decline in income is mainly due to the continuing decline in reimbursement by Medicare and private insurers. Usually this impacts primary care specialties that rely on office visits, more than other medical specialties that are procedure oriented.

Building Block #5

Burn out among Pediatric Oncologists, one of the toughest specialties in medicine.

Pediatric Blood Cancer. 2011 Dec 15;57(7):1168-73. doi: 10.1002/pbc.23121. Epub 2011 May 5.

Career burnout among pediatric oncologists.

Roth M1, Morrone K, Moody K, Kim M, Wang D, Moadel A, Levy A.

A study published in Pediatric Blood & Cancer in 2011 attempted to find out how working in a specialty that deals with life-threatening illnesses affects the chances of developing burnout syndrome. A survey included the 22 questions of Maslach Burnout Inventory, as well as questions regarding work-related and lifestyle-related factors associated with developing burn- out.

A total of 1047 practicing pediatric oncologists were surveyed, of those 410 responded (40%) to the survey.

72% had at least moderate levels of burnout

38% had high levels of burnout

Women had a higher burnout rate of 47% comparable to 32% of

male pediatric oncologists.

Physicians in practice less than 10 years had a higher rate of burnout of 50% comparable to 33% for those who have been in practice for more than 10 years.

Physicians who reported satisfaction with their lives outside of work were less likely to experience burnout

Availability of a forum for debriefing and services for physicians affected by burnout were both associated with lower rates of burnout, at a rate of 24%, compared to 46% of those who did not have these avenues available to them.

Only 36% of respondents reported their institutions had a forum for debriefing.

Only 40% of the respondents reported their institutions had services available to physicians experiencing symptoms of burnout.

The paper concluded that approximately ¾ of pediatric oncologists experience burnout.

Building Block #6

Pediatric intensivists vs. general pediatricians in Brazil

Pediatric Research (2010)

Burnout Syndrome Among Pediatricians: A Case Control Study Comparing Pediatric Intensivists and General Pediatricians

R G Branco1, T T Garcia2, M E Molon2, P C R Garcia3, J P Piva3 and P E Ferreira4

1Paediatrics, Cambridge University, Cambridge, UK

2Department of Pediatrics, Pontificia Universidad Católica do Rio Grande do Sul, Porto Alegre, Brazil

3Paediatric Intensive Care Unit, Hospital Sao Lucas da PUCRS, Porto Alegre, Brazil

4Department of Psychiatry, Pontificia Universidad Católica do Rio Grande do Sul, Porto Alegre, Brazil

Burnout was present in 71% of the PICU group and in 29% of the General Pediatric group.

The paper concluded that burnout among pediatric intensivists is frequent and characteristically manifested by high levels of emotional exhaustion, depersonalization and low levels of professional accomplishment. These characteristics suggest a low quality of life, emotional suffering and professional dissatisfaction.

Building Block #7

American Academy of Pediatrics study: Pediatrician Life and Career Experience (PLACES)

Predictors of burn-out Results from the Pediatrician Life and Career Experience Study (PLACES)

Mary Pat Frintner, MSPH,1 Amy J Starmer, MD, MPH2, 3

1Research, American Academy of Pediatrics, Elk Grove, United States; 2Doernbecher Children's Hospital, Oregon Health and Science University, Portland, United States; 3Boston Children's Hospital, Boston, United States

93% of PLACES participants completed the survey.

84% reported satisfaction with their career.

28% reported current burnout in their work.

In multivariable analyses, poor balance between personal and professional commitments and hectic work setting were the strongest predictors of burnout.

Those currently in general pediatrics or hospitalist positions were more likely to report burnout than those in subspecialty positions. Pediatricians who report working more years in their current job, more hours per week and those less satisfied with their career also reported more burnout.

Building Block #8

Psychiatrists, what is the deal?

Logically, psychiatry is a career which lends itself to a high burnout rate. However, surprisingly many published papers and articles rate psychiatry as experiencing some of the lowest burnout rates in the medical profession. One of the characteristics of modern psychiatrists is that they do not take Medicare or Medicaid, and for that matter many of the insurances which do not pay well. This may help to reduce the stress of being in practice today.

Building Block #9

"Secular Priest" burn out is higher than "Religious Priests" burn out in India

What the heck!!!!!!!

How this could be related to medicine!!!!!!!

Does this have anything to do with the Hippocratic Oath!!!!!

Pastoral Psychology

November 2005, Volume 54, Issue 2, pp 157-171

Burnout and Depression Among Catholic Priests in India

Antony Raj,

Karol E. Dean

This study examined burnout and depression among Catholic priests in Southern India using the Maslach Burnout Inventory and the Center for Epidemiological Studies -Depression scale (Robinson, Shaver, & Wrightsman, 1991). Additionally, a demographic survey assessing four predictor variables was administered. The participants included 50 secular priests and 51 religious priests randomly selected from two dioceses. The study found that diocesan/secular priests experienced significantly more burnout and depression than did religious order priests. This indicates that structural and administrative systems can lead to burnout and depression. The findings of this investigation would be of help for priests in both the United States and in India to identify problems, encourage reorientation of their lives towards the spiritual, and to promote emotional maturity.

So with some stretch of imagination, and in a completely non-scientific, totally opinionated way, we attempt to stimulate you to think about the subject rather than simply accept our explanation and justification. We abstract that medicine is an art and science with a higher moral commitment to patients' well-being that is parallel to the commitment of religious leaders. This is what physicians have sworn to do through the "Hippocratic Oath". If our assumption is true, then we can learn something about higher burnout rates from this study because its observations indicate that structural and administrative systems can lead to burnout and depression.

Building Block #10

Using the same assumption that physicians are art-practicing scientists with a high moral commitment to their patients' health, parallel to religious leaders, we tap into this study on Catholic priests' burnout. We will leave you to your own conclusions about this study and how to benefit from it in your own journey of self-exploration.

Burnout in Catholic clergy: A predictive model using psychological and spiritual variables.

Rossetti, Stephen J.; Rhoades, Colin J.

Psychology of Religion and Spirituality, Vol 5(4), Nov 2013, 335-341

Catholic priests are faced with innumerable demands, unrealistic expectations, and few tangible results. Moreover, in today's society, there are fewer priests, even greater demands, and a surrounding culture that is increasingly secular and apparently less supportive. Thus, burnout in Catholic clergy is commonly presumed to be high.

The purpose of this study was to move beyond assumptions and explore the real extent of burnout among Roman Catholic clergy (using a standardized test of burnout) and then to explore those variables that were statistically related to burnout. A sample of 2,482 Catholic priests across the United States is given the Maslach Burnout Inventory. They scored significantly less burned out than Maslach Burnout Inventory norm groups that included a general sample and that also included those who were male or who worked in social services or medicine.

When investigating those variables that were associated with burnout, exercise and taking time off were significantly correlated to lower levels of burnout; however, the effect was small. The more important variables associated with burnout were job satisfaction, inner peace, childhood psychological problems, relationship to God, and good friends. On these more important variables, priests reported high levels of health and well-being.

A large majority indicated being happy as priests and reported having good friendships, satisfaction with their relationship to God, a limited history of childhood psychological problems, and a strong sense of inner peace. For Catholic priests, and likely for all people, strong psychological and spiritual support systems seem to be most important in preventing burnout, especially for those engaged in the demanding positions of caring for others.

Building Block #11

Stress induces structural changes in the brain.

Kaufer and colleagues, Journal of Molecular Psychiatry published Feb. 11, 2014

Kaufer and colleagues from the University of Berkley published an article in the Journal of Molecular Psychiatry on Feb. 11, 2014, showing that chronic stress generates long-term changes in the brain that may explain why people suffering chronic stress are prone to mental problems such as anxiety and mood disorders later in life.

In a series of experiments, Daniela Kaufer, UC Berkeley associate professor of integrative biology, and her colleagues, discovered that chronic stress generates more myelin-producing cells and fewer neurons than normal. This results in an excess of myelin – and thus, white matter – in some areas of the brain, which disrupts the delicate balance and timing of communication within the brain.

A theorized possible mechanism emerged utilizing this particular discovery. It may shed some light on, and help to explain, changes in brain connectivity in people with Post Traumatic Stress Disorder (PTSD). For example, those patients could develop more white matter connections between the Hippocampus and the Amygdala, and fewer connections between Hippocampus and prefrontal cortex. Amygdala is involved in responses to fear, fight and flight, while prefrontal cortex regulates our response.

In theory, more connections to the more primitive responses of fear and fight dominated by the Amygdala, will mean faster response than the less connected prefrontal cortex where responses can be dampened. So in this pathologic state, and when stress in induced, the inhibitory prefrontal pathways do not work as fast as the Amygdala, thereby sending more "scary and alarming" signals.

Kaufer's lab, which conducts research on the molecular and cellular effects of acute and chronic stress, focused in this study on neural stem cells in the hippocampus of the brains of adult rats. These stem cells were previously thought to mature only into neurons or a type of glial cell called an astrocyte. The researchers found, however, that chronic stress also made stem cells in the hippocampus mature into another type of glial cell called an oligodendrocyte, which produces the myelin that sheaths nerve cells.

The finding, which they demonstrated in rats and cultured rat brain cells, suggests a key role for oligodendrocytes in long-term and perhaps permanent changes in the brain that could set the stage for later mental problems. Oligodendrocytes also help form synapses – sites where one cell talks to another – and help control the growth pathway of axons, which make those synapse connections.

The fact that chronic stress also decreases the number of stem cells that mature into neurons could provide an explanation for how chronic stress also affects learning and memory, said Kaufer.

Kaufer is now conducting experiments to determine how stress in infancy affects the brain's white matter, and whether chronic early-life stress decreases resilience later in life. She also is looking at the effects of therapies, ranging from exercise to antidepressant drugs, which reduce the impact of stress and stress hormones.

Building Block #12

Burnout During Residency Training

Journal of graduate medical education. 2009 Dec; 1(2): 236–242.

doi: 10.4300/JGME-D-09-00054.1

PMCID: PMC2931238

Burnout During Residency Training: A Literature Review

Waguih William IsHak, MD, FAPA, Sara Lederer, PsyD, Carla Mandili, MD, Rose Nikravesh, DO, Laurie Seligman, MA, Monisha Vasa, MD, Dotun Ogunyemi, MD, and Carol A. Bernstein, MD

In this literature review, examination of the burnout literature reveals that it is:

28%–45% among medical students

27-75% among residents, depending on specialty

The paper states that distress during medical school can lead to burnout, which in turn can result in negative consequences as a working physician. Burnout also poses significant challenges during early training years in residency. Time demands, lack of control, work planning, work organization, inherently difficult job situations, and interpersonal relationships are all considered factors that contribute to residents' burnout.

Potential interventions include workplace-driven and individual-driven measures. Workplace interventions include education about burnout, workload modifications, increasing the diversity of work duties, stress management training, mentoring, emotional intelligence training, and wellness workshops. Individual-driven behavioral, social, and physical activities include promoting interpersonal professional relations, meditation, counseling, and exercise.

The paper further concludes that educators need to develop an active awareness of burnout and ought to consider incorporating relevant instruction and interventions during the process of training resident physicians.

Building Block #13

Maslach Burnout Inventory

You have been hearing about frequently. What is it?

The Maslach Burnout Inventory (MBI) is the most commonly used questionnaire in research studies to measure burnout. The MBI human services survey is a self-administered, 22-item questionnaire that was developed to measure burnout in human services workers and is regarded to be the "gold standard" in measuring burnout.

The MBI items are rated on a Likert scale from 0 to 6 (0 = never, 1 = a few times per year, 2 = once a month, 3 = a few times per month, 4 = once a week, 5 = a few times per week, and 6 = every day) and score sample items such as: "I feel emotionally drained from my work." It is designed to assess the 3 primary dimensions of burnout: emotional exhaustion, depersonalization, and personal accomplishment.

Burnout is detected using cutoff scores of high emotional exhaustion ($\geq$27), high depersonalization ($\geq$10), and low personal accomplishment ($\leq$33), based on normative data from 1104 medical professionals.

Many studies using the MBI define burnout as high emotional exhaustion or depersonalization. The personal accomplishment scores are less commonly included because they are thought to correlate less with psychological strain.

Building Block #14

From Hungry; female physicians, burnout, and reproductive health

Reproductive health and burn-out among female physicians: nationwide, representative study from Hungary

Zsuzsa Győrffy1*, Diána Dweik2 and Edmond Girasek3

*Corresponding author: Zsuzsa Győrffy gyorffy@chello.hu

Author Affiliations

1Institute of Behavioural Sciences, Semmelweis University, Nagyvárad square 4, H-1089 Budapest, Hungary

2Department of Obstetrics and Gynecology, University of Szeged, Semmelweis st. 1Szeged, H-6725 Szeged, Hungary

3Health Services Management Training Centre, Semmelweis University, Kútvölgyi st 2, 1125 Budapest, Hungary

For all author emails, please log on.

BMC Women's Health 2014, 14:121 doi:10.1186/1472-6874-14-121

The electronic version of this article is the complete one and can be found online at:http://www.biomedcentral.com/1472-6874/14/121

This study compared female physicians to the general female population in Hungry.

1- Female physicians were more often characterized by time-to-pregnancy interval longer than one year 18.4%, compared to 9.8% for the general female population.

2- Female physicians were bearing more high-risk pregnancies 26.3%, compared to 16.3% for the general female population.

3- Female physicians were more likely to be undergoing infertility therapy 8.5%, compared to 3.4% of the general female population.

4- Female physicians were experiencing miscarriage at a rate of 20.8%, compared to 14.6% of the general female population during their reproductive years.

5- With the exception of miscarriages, the difference remained significant in all comparisons within the professional control group.

6- Both high-risk pregnancies and miscarriages experienced by doctors were associated with depersonalization ($p = 0.028$ and $p = 0.012$ respectively) and personal accomplishment ($p = 0.016$ and $p = 0.008$ respectively) dimensions of burnout.

7- Results of the multivariate analysis showed that, besides traditional risk factors, depersonalization acted as an important explanatory factor in case of high-risk pregnancies ($OR = 1.086$).

The paper authors concluded that there is a circulatory causality between burnout and the development of reproductive disorders. Burnout is an important risk factor for high-risk pregnancies and miscarriages, and it has a negative effect on the outcome of pregnancies. At the same time, women suffering from reproductive disorders are more likely to develop burnout syndrome.

Improvement of working conditions and prevention of burnout in female doctors are equally important tasks in addressing these findings.

Building Block #15

Prevalence and predictors of burnout among specialty palliative care clinicians in the United States: Results of a national survey.

This paper is presented in the

2014 Palliative Care in Oncology Symposium

General Poster Session B: Early Integration of Palliative Care in Cancer Care, Patient-Reported Outcomes, and Psycho-Oncology
Oral Abstract Session B: Early Integration of Palliative Care, Burnout Issues, and Mindfulness

Abstract Number: 87

Citation: J Clin Oncol 32, 2014 (suppl 31; abstr 87)

Author(s):

Arif Kamal, Janet Bull, Steven Wolf, Greg Samsa, Katherine Ast, Keith Mark Swetz, Tait D. Shanafelt, Amy Pickar Abernethy; Duke University Medical Center, Durham, NC; Four Seasons Hospice, Flat Rock, NC; American Academy of Hospice and Palliative Medicine, Chicago, IL; Mayo Clinic, Rochester, MN

This study was not unique to physicians and it included, for example, advanced practice providers, registered nurses and chaplains who were all members of the American Academy of Hospice and Palliative Medicine.

The Maslach Burnout Inventory (MBI) was used to determine

burnout severity across two domains, emotional exhaustion and depersonalization.

Severity is reported as "low", "moderate", or "high".

"High" is consistent with burnout.

A total of 1,241 clinicians responded to the survey, which represents approximately 30% of the clinicians contacted.

- 68% of respondents were physicians.
- 57% of the respondents were over age 50
- 65% were females
- 82% were married or partnered
- 67% had worked in the field for less than 10 years.
- 42% took overnight call regularly
- 30% reported working 50 hours per week or more
- 57% had at least 4 colleagues
- 24% reported high depersonalization, one of the components of burn-out
- 59% reported high emotional exhaustion
- 62% of reported high burnout symptoms on either emotional exhaustion or depersonalization scales.

The clinicians at the greatest risk for burnout were:

1- Younger physicians
2- Those working more than 50 hours per week
3- Those with fewer colleagues within their practice

Building Block #16

Loss of autonomy

"Freidson" has been identified for the last two decades as the leading theorist on professional autonomy. He has recently defined autonomy in the following manner:

Taken as an ideal type, complete autonomy is sustained by an occupational monopoly embracing several dimensions. It is first of all an economic monopoly: the profession controls recruitment, training, and credentialing so it can regulate directly the number of practitioners available to meet demand. This has obvious implications for income. Economic monopoly is viable, however, because professional autonomy also includes a political monopoly over an area of expertise; the profession is accepted as the authoritative spokesman on affairs related to its body of knowledge and skill, and so its representatives serve as expert guides for legislation and administrative rules bearing on its work. Furthermore, the profession has an administrative or supervisory monopoly over the practical affairs connected with its work; its members fill the organizational ranks which are concerned with establishing work standards, directing and evaluating work. "Peer review" rather than hierarchical directive is the norm. Clearly as I have defined it, professional autonomy represents a privileged position of some significance (Freidson, 1994).

We are going to try to translate this into real life issues. With that in mind we are going to divide autonomy of physicians into two categories:

- Financial autonomy
- Clinical autonomy

Financial autonomy has been eroded with physicians' voluntary decision to exchange more financial security for less financial autonomy. They did that first by participating in Medicare, and then by negotiating private insurance contracts. Because physicians do not have real negotiating power, payers have managed to continue to slash their fees.

The **clinical autonomy** of practicing medicine has been a real moral dilemma in the medical community. Physicians are not able to adapt as easily as other professionals to the concept of the "bottom line".

One of the examples of this is the high burnout rate among medical directors who make decisions on behalf of insurance carriers on whether to deny or authorize medical diagnostic studies or procedures.

Building Block #17

Investment into medical education and return on this investment

For this subject we cite the abstract of a paper published by Nicolas Roth- UC Berkley by the title:

The Costs and Returns on Medical Education:

"By treating medical school tuition payments and the opportunity costs of foregone wages as investments in human capital. I calculated the internal rates of return and the net present values of those investments across a range of medical specialties. I calculate these values under two different sets of assumptions. I also use two different discount rates to calculate net present values.

Radiation oncologists, radiologists, and orthopedic surgeons enjoy the greatest returns on their investments, while rheumatologists, general pediatricians, and endocrinologist experience the lowest returns.

I also find physician median earnings to be very good predictors of net present values. It is not clear whether physicians experience increasing, decreasing, or steady returns to scale for investments in additional years of residency training. An analysis of physicians who sub-specialize may help to answer this question. "

Building Block #18

Intuitive understanding that a patient's health will continue to decline

I write very little under this category. When your patient is deathly ill, as a physician you know it, no matter what the labs, radiology studies, and other data say otherwise.

Building Block #19

Evidence Based Medicine

I am going to be very conservative touching on this subject. I understand it is an extremely sensitive issue, especially when many regulatory bodies have been pushing very hard for using more evidence based medicine. As you have noticed in the majority of my writings, I am actually fans of evidence based medicine. However, there is growing frustration among physicians with using it. Just Google the subject on your own and you will hear the voices of many frustrated physicians.

Of all the concerns in health care today, we have elected to list the following as contributing to burnout. I do not know if this is scientifically proven or not, but it is a source of frustration to many practicing physicians, which is another variable in the development of Burnout syndrome:

1- Evidence based medicine is being promoted by insurance companies to limit access to expensive procedures.

2- Evidence based medicine covers only 20% of the medicine practiced.

3- Many of the studies are not large enough, or reliable enough.

4- Evidence based medicine is sometimes ambiguous.

Overall I feel that evidence based medicine has been serving patients and physicians very well. It becomes a problem when administrative entities use it rigidly and indiscriminately. Then it immediately becomes perceived by physicians as interference with practicing medicine, infringement on clinical autonomy, and depersonalization of care.

In general, my guess is that physicians use evidence based medicine as a guide line for practicing more educated medicine, like they have been doing for thousands of years. While number crunchers use evidence based medicine in a more rigid way, a formula where 1+1=2 always.

Building Block #20

The difficult doctor

This is an article published in the British Medical Journal Health Services in 2006 that attempted to explore the characteristics of physicians who report frustration with patients.

BMC Health Serv Res. 2006 Oct 6;6:128.

The difficult doctor? Characteristics of physicians who report frustration with patients: an analysis of survey data.

Krebs EE1, Garrett JM, Konrad TR.

In this study a secondary analysis was conducted using the Physicians Worklife Survey. This survey included 1391 physicians of the following specialties: family medicine, general internal medicine, and medicine subspecialties. The survey assessed physician and practice characteristics, including stress, depression and anxiety symptoms, practice setting, work hours, case-mix, and control over administrative and clinical practice.

Physicians estimated the percentage of their patients who were "generally frustrating to deal with." Then the researchers categorized physicians by quartile of reported frustrating patients and compared characteristics of physicians in the top quartile to those in the other three quartiles.

Results of the adjusted analysis are:

Physicians who reported high frustration with patients were:

1- Younger

2- Worked more hours per week

3- Had more symptoms of depression, stress, and anxiety

Factors independently associated with high frustration included:

1- Age < 40 years

2- Work hours > 55 per week

3- Higher stress.

4- Practice in a medicine subspecialty.

5- Greater number of patients with psychosocial problems or substance abuse.

The researchers concluded that personal and practice characteristics of physicians who report high frustration with patients differ from those of other physicians.

A Road Map

So far you have developed your own opinion about possible causes of burnout syndrome, no matter what stage you may be in. With the following list, we attempt to further stimulate your brain in exploring more possible etiologies of the burnout phenomenon. These brain-thinking stimulators are not listed according to importance, because "most important" varies among physicians, specialties, and type of practice:

1- Increased administrative duties

2- Long work hours

3- Changing health care environment, uncertainty and lack of predictability. One of the most interesting examples of lack of logic in this whole process is the Medicare fee schedule. Every year the congress has to pass a law to prevent the enactment of the law passed a few years back to slash Medicare fees by about 50%

4- Declining income, more pronounced in cognitive specialties.

5- Growing unpaid services; the physician cannot afford not to provide care to be able to maintain quality medicine, because they cannot be categorized under face-face contact.

6- Lack of professional fulfillment

7- Lack of satisfaction with the level of care being delivered to patients due to insurance or employer restraints.

8-Too many difficult patients in the daily schedule, as simple straight forward problems get shifted to mid-levels. These "easy" cases are critical to create a variety of case load throughout the work day.

9- EMRs are a burden; the technology is tailored toward tracking services. What physicians need is EMRs that can help them deliver services.

10-Untrained corporate managers who are in charge of managing physicians. The best example to describe this situation is as follows; hiring very experienced gamers on "Call of Duty" to be actual commanders in a real-life battle field leading a unit into a real-life dangerous neighborhood. They have never seen explosions with splattered bodies; they never had to sooth a dying person. They have only seen and experienced that in the virtual gaming world. They have no clue of what physicians do, but because they have to lead, it is learning on the job. Who pays the heftiest price for that education? Usually physicians!

The number of inexperienced managers responsible for physician supervision is increasing, as smaller and medium size hospitals try to grow unrealistically into World Class Clinics. With that in mind, we remind those of you who do not know about Mayo Clinic, a real World Class Clinic, about how they manage their physicians. In summary, a department chairman, who is usually a well-accomplished and published physician in their own specialty, is chosen every 4-5 years. After the end of his/her term the chief goes back to being part of the front line team. His/her administrative duties are supported by a non-medical manager usually with an MBA in business.

11- Not enough time to relax

12- Not enough time to exercise

13- Not enough time to sleep

14-Unbalanced life/work

15-Conflicts and tension at work with the ancillary staff; a situation in which physicians have no say beyond filing complaints. A great example of this is when a sub-standard medical assistant doesn't meet the requisite level of specific physician productivity and care standards and needs to be relieved of duty. It can be months before a replacement is offered to the physician. Meanwhile the "numbers" of the physician will suffer for each quarterly "practice parameter" that managers use to assess each physician. On top of that, the problem for the physician will be tremendous frustration and feeling a total "lack of control" while the big system tries to respond appropriately, but usually slowly, to the grievances.

16- Too little time for patients on the schedule for a meaningful visit.

17- Too many patients on the schedule

3 TAKING THE FUN OUT OF PRACTICING MEDICINE

Remember the days when you couldn't wait to practice medicine? You spent countless hours studying to become the best physician you could be, because you were going to heal people. Your passion carried you through the years of schooling, internships and residencies until you were able to practice on your own. What happened to that motivation? Where did your energy go? When did the fun of practicing medicine evaporate?

At the heart of each physician is the desire to help patients. When the time spent with patients is impacted by uncontrollable business pressures, so is the self-satisfaction and pride that once came with the job. These are the first smoldering dissatisfactions that can eventually lead to Burnout syndrome. If practicing medicine is no longer fun for you, ask yourself why.

- Is it because of too many administrative burdens?
- It is because of revenue pressures?

- Is it because you simply want to work with patients and not run a business?

OR

Is practicing medicine no longer fun because you no longer have the motivation, the interest and the engagement in the practice of your specialty?

If you answered yes to the last question, do yourself a great favor and consider that you may be headed for Burnout syndrome. An increasing number of your colleagues are suffering silently with Burnout because the symptoms, considered individually, can easily be dismissed as something else- a cold, lack of time off, short staff, or age. That's part of the problem; the symptoms of burnout when considered *collectively* are the best, and only, diagnosis.

Who Is The Medical Student

The medical student is you many years ago. It is important we take you back to those days and remind you of who you were.

(These characteristics are not unique to medical students; students pursuing other professions list some of these as their motivations as well.)

Think back to when you were in medical school, full of passion and enthusiasm for your studies and your career. You probably would have said you have many of the characteristics listed below.

However, as you now know, having some or even a majority of these characteristics is not enough to get a student through medical school, residency, and a career as a physician. The pressure is too great, the hours too long, for empathy alone to see you through.

Furthermore, the majority of medical students are 22-24 years old, an age where most of students at colleges at that age are still exploring their right fit in the world. Instead, the average medical student is studying, working and researching all day every day, just to keep their place in the student body.

How many of these characteristics do you remember having when you began your studies in medicine?

- Empathy
- The nag- does this mean urge? to help
- The satisfaction from helping others
- The desire to make a difference
- The satisfaction that comes from making a difference in people's lives
- The desire to explore
- The satisfaction of finding a solution
- The motivation to put personnel needs on hold
- The determination to see difficult projects through
- The motivation to excel
- The satisfaction of accomplishment
- The comfort in functioning with complete autonomy

- The satisfaction of being autonomous
- The comfort with making the difficult call
- The comfort with making the final call
- The satisfaction of making the final call
- The comfort and satisfaction of being the ship's captain
- The need for recognition
- The satisfaction of peer recognition
- The need for prestige, the type that money and popularity cannot achieve
- Self-confidence
- The ability to grow
- Financial security

The Happy Practice

This is our own due diligence and is not supported by any paper or article. We believe these characteristics are the pillars of a happy practice that fosters the best atmosphere for having fun practicing medicine.

1- Autonomy
2- Utilization decisions are made in response to lack of funds or resources rather than being based on recommendations according to profit margins.
3- Satisfying patient-physician encounters

There are many other variables that can affect the practice of medicine. However, we believe that if physicians do not perceive the critical importance of the 3 aforementioned pillars remaining intact, none of the other variables will be sufficient to maintain the fun in practicing medicine.

We suggest that "Losing fun practicing medicine" is the very critical turning point in a physician's career and a strong predictor of developing high rates of burnout in a medical practice. Of course this concept has yet to be proven by a scientific study.

Why this is a very important concept?

Because if it is accepted or proven as accurate, it may lead to a radical change in the way practices, large health care organizations, and CEOs approach the pressing issue of Burnout.

I think that CEOs should start using the one item question "Are You Still Having Fun Practicing Medicine in Our Group?" as a screening tool for physicians' burnout, rather than using "Maslach Burnout Inventory BMI" with its 22 questions.

Although I do not have any research to support this claim, I think it is a sensitive predictor, in the very early stages of burnout symptoms, of potential full-blown burnout among physicians in a practice group.

Nearly 45% of physicians in practice today report that they are exhausted from too many administrative tasks, saying they are "burned out". Seventy percent of physicians say they spend more than one day a week on paperwork when they would rather be spending time with their patients. It's a catch-22 really. If you don't spend time on paperwork you won't submit timely billings; but if you don't spend time with patients, you won't have any time to bill. It doesn't take a lot of imagination to understand why many physicians feel the fun of practicing medicine is long gone.

Burnout syndrome takes the fun out of your work, and your life overall. In order to address it you first have to recognize it, so let's talk in detail about how burnout can destroy the happiness and self-satisfaction you used to derive from practicing medicine.

Janis Finer, MD[1], a primary-care physician in Tulsa, Okla., is a good example of what burnout can do. The Washington Post told her story in an article about physician burnout in 2014 and it is worth relating here. According to the Post, Dr. Finer gave up her busy practice at the age of 57 to become a hospitalist because she wanted to work regular shifts, have some time off and get an increase in pay. Before she left her practice to become a hospitalist, Dr. Finer had become tired of the business side of running a practice and sold her practice to a hospital. The Post story reports that it didn't help. Hospital administrators told her she needed to see 22 to 28 patients a day. "At one point, we were scheduled to see patients every 11 minutes," Finer said.

According to a survey conducted by Medscape, 45% of female physicians report suffering from burnout while 37% of male physicians report suffering from the syndrome. It may be that women are more willing to openly admit they are burned out, or it may be that they tend to practice in family medicine and Ob/Gyn which are two of the highest stress areas of medicine (along with emergency medicine).

The website www.mommmd.com was created to "encourage and support women physicians, residents," and other female clinicians in their careers, and personal life. The site's discussion forum is full of female physicians trying to find a way to avoid professional burnout or, leave medicine altogether. The posts are anonymous which tends to encourage candid posts. They are important to share:

"I see close to 60 people a day in my ob-gyn practice. Don't ask how I do it because at the end of the day, my head is swirling. I do this because that is the only way I can make my overhead and actually take home enough to pay for the nanny and student loans. It is ridiculous."

"To survive burnout, you have to prioritize exactly what is important to you. Career, family, free time, community involvement, research, or whatever. You may need to quit your current job and look for one which is more compatible to the lifestyle you want and need to have. Take some time off and don't work at all, things may start to fall into place then, once all the stressors have been relieved. Just remember, you're not the only one in burnout phase."

Another post says: "Alternative options within the medical profession are out there, even if difficult to find. I really struggled to find something that I could get by with. So, I wound up in urgent care. It's a great job in terms of hours and lifestyle. Extremely low stress and I work "full time" which is 36 hours per week (three 12-hour days), about half of what I was working before and less than I'd have worked doing part-time at my other job. No call, no nights, no rounds, only one weekend a month. The pay is considerably less than my full-time family practice job, but considerably more than anywhere I looked into for part-time work (and fewer hours of actual work than the "part-time" family practice jobs). I have a fairly happy life now. I'm content and my family is happy and healthy and functioning. We are expecting our third child in January, something that would never have happened in my previous career path."

Former internist Diane Shannon wrote a column for Boston's National Public Radio (NPR) station's website column "Commonwealth Health",[4] entitled "Why I Left Medicine: A Burntout Doctor's Decision to Quit". In it she says, "I no longer remembered the joy I'd felt when I first began medical school, and I couldn't imagine surviving life as a doctor." She went on to describe the physical and mental symptoms she was suffering that led to her exit from medical practice.

"As an internist, working in adult outpatient clinics around Boston, I had trouble leaving my work at work. I'd go for a run and spend the entire 30 minutes wondering if I'd ordered the right diagnostic test. I suffered from chronic early morning wakening, even on my weekends off. I startled easily. I found it impossible to relax. I worried constantly that I'd make a mistake, like ordering the wrong dosage of a medication, or that a system flaw, like an abnormal lab report getting overlooked, would harm a patient."

Some researchers are concerned that burnout syndrome is being treated as a psychological disease, rather than the result of a broken, dysfunctional healthcare system. When asked why they have become dissatisfied with practicing medicine, the top reasons stated by physicians certainly point to the healthcare system. The top 5 reasons given in the Medscape survey, born out in numerous other studies as well, include:

- Too many bureaucratic tasks
- Spending too many hours at work
- Impact of the Affordable Care Act
- Feeling like a cog in the wheel
- Income not high enough

As Diane Shannon wrote, "I was less immune than others to the stresses of practicing medicine in a health care system that often seemed blind to humanness, both mine and my patients'."

If you no longer enjoy practicing medicine, don't try to talk yourself out of it. That is one of the first signs that you are heading toward full-fledged burnout. Losing your passion for the work is serious. It can lead to medical mistakes, and physical illness for you, the physician, as a recent survey showed.

A study published in Anesthesia and Analgesia reported that one-third of 1500 anesthesiology residents who scored high for burnout and depression risk reported multiple medication errors during the last year, compared with less than 1% of the residents at lower risk. Forty-one percent of those residents demonstrated high risk of burnout and 22% demonstrated a high risk of depression. High risk of both burnout and depression occurred in 17% of residents.

Despite the burnout and depression caused by practicing medicine, many doctors report feeling trapped in their chosen careers. A post on mommd.com says, "Most of the doctors I know are frustrated being in the profession. Many would leave if they found a way to support their current lifestyles. Most are so locked into their earnings that they cannot conceive of leaving medicine, despite the unhappiness. It's a shame."

Money is a very real consideration when considering whether or not to change your career. However, burnout is serious enough to warrant changing your lifestyle. Numerous studies show that burnout and the associated depression leads to a higher suicide rate in US physicians. That is a game changer. Burnout is powerful- and preventing it is worth changing your life, adjusting how you practice medicine, or changing your career completely.

For a bit of brevity, it might help to consider the wise words of one famous "doctor" known for his fun take on life. In fact, he probably has done more to convey the wisdom of life through silliness than anyone else. This "doctor" is Dr. Seuss. Here is what he had to say about the fleeting nature of time, and life.

"How did it get so late so soon? Its night before its afternoon. December is here before its June. My goodness how the time has flown. How did it get so late so soon?"

Burnout Syndrome hates fun, self-satisfaction and motivation. Here are some of the ways it accomplishes that:

Working Harder

The second most common reason for feeling burned out is spending too many hours at work. This would indicate that physicians are working longer hours to get the work done, and to find a feeling of satisfaction in their work again. When work is not the right fit, working harder becomes the norm, and is a result of setting higher personal expectations. That is where the snowball effect begins; higher expectations are set, so more time is spent working to meet the higher bar, more time is spent completing tasks, and less time is spent enjoying life. This may gradually escalate to the point where time devoted to completing work is favored at the expense of friends, family, eating, and sleeping time. Where is the joy in that?

A: If less patient time reduces the self-fulfillment you have always gained from your practice, then you may begin to work harder. After all, won't more hours in the day give you more chance to prove yourself to you?

Do you feel this way?   Few times a week / daily / most of the time

If you think about it candidly, do you feel that you are neglecting your own needs?   Few times a week / daily / most of the time

Denial of Emerging Problems

Irritability, sarcasm, and more aggression is seen from the viewpoint of outside observers.

There is some self-awareness that something is wrong, but there is difficulty identifying the reason. This is when the first physical symptoms may start to manifest themselves. Emotions start to become blunt. Avoidance and isolationism start to become more of an issue.

A: Is there no fun in practicing medicine because you don't feel well? Every day seems to involve numerous problems; many more than there used to be. It seems as though the only way to run the practice is to be tough with the staff. Any visitors except patients are told to go away, and even hospital or group administration has to wait to see you. You realize that you seem unable to have fun, both in your professional and personal life, but you can't figure out why.

Do you feel this way?   Few times a week / daily / most of the time

There is No Use Trying

Burnout is characterized by decreased mental energy, absenteeism, and reduced job satisfaction. One can feel a lack of hope with the work path one is on, depression can set in.

A: Have you felt a low level of personal accomplishment for a while? It's difficult to get motivated to go to work every day. For some reason you would rather lie around the house in your pajamas, watching reality TV, something you never dreamt would happen to you. You don't see any way to improve your practice, or to get out of the practice and do something different. It's all just one big hopeless mess and there is no way out. You are beginning to eat more and drink more, more frequently.

Do you feel this way?   Few times a week / daily / most of the time

As you leave this chapter, remember the words of Dr. Seuss:

You have brains in your head. You have feet in your shoes. You

can steer yourself in any direction you choose. You're on your own, and you know what you know. And you are the guy who'll decide where to go.

Dr. Seuss

The good news is that fun is a good way to treat burnout syndrome. There are other effective treatments as well and we will talk about them in later chapters. Just know that infusing your life with fun is a good thing.

Resources:

1. http://**www.washingtonpost.com**/national/health-science/a-growing-number-of-primary-care-doctors-are-burning-out-how-does-this-affect-patients/2014/03/31/2e8bce24-a951-11e3-b61e-8051b8b52d06_story.html

2. http://**commonhealth.wbur.org**/2013/10/why-i-left-medicine-a-burnt-out-doctors-decision-to-quit

3. http://**www.mommd.com**/givingup.shtml

4. http://**www.medscape.com**/features/slideshow/lifestyle/2013/public#4

5. http://**www.brainyquote.com**/quotes/authors/d/dr_seuss.html#IQV3Psr8D1K4zjsY.99

6. http://**www.kevinmd.com**/blog/2013/08/burnout-perfect-storm-physician-stress.html

4 THE ROOTS

I have formulated my own theory and opinion about the roots of burnout syndrome among physicians. In this chapter I try to explain how it is possible for a very competitive, hard-working, dedicated, passionate, focused physician who loves taking care of people, and who has proven him or herself to be resilient from the first day of medical school to the first day of practice, suddenly begins to slide into the burnout path only 3 to 5 years into their career.

Many well respected authors, psychologists, organizations and legislative bodies may look down on our conclusions. This book is not written for them, it is written for you, the physician who knows that there is something really wrong and you are searching for a light to help you find your way. This chapter will hand you a flashlight with one intensely focused beam that will reveal the path to you. You will have to walk around and explore life for yourself, but I will give you the light to help to reveal the truth.

I will present you with a constellation of concepts from which you can develop your own conclusions. They are presented in an orderly, sequential fashion, but feel free to read them in any order you like.

Working Harder and the Compulsion to Prove Oneself

I do not claim to know for sure that my following observations are true and applicable to all physicians who are suffering from burnout. Indeed, I believe that there is dire need for a scientific, measurable study, one that can be replicated, to assess the dimensions of this stage of burnout. Why is it critical? Because it seems that the "working harder and the compulsion to prove oneself" is the stage where the cascade of burnout symptoms- the chain reaction of one sign leading to the next, begins. Discovering the trigger to this chain reaction would be the key to a fundamental solution for preventing burnout syndrome, rather than fragmented articles here and there, the isolated attempts like this self-help book by us, and non-comprehensive writings about the subject.

When you have the chance to review the current writings on burnout syndrome among physicians, they will give you the impression that this epidemic is a psychological one, more or less a sub-type of depression. I think about it more like an action-reaction phenomena in its early stages that can evolve quickly into a psychological-like condition.

The initial trigger is purely extrinsic and could be one or all of the following:

1- Moral mismatch

2- Economic mismatch

3- Intellectual mismatch

The product of any of these mismatches between the physician and the practice is usually negative feelings. Whenever faced with negative feelings, the natural response is to avoid them, and the simplest way to cope is to walk away from the triggers of negativity. The problem is that this is frequently not possible for physicians; not only because changing practice or employment is a lengthy process and can easily take up to 2 years; but mainly because finding options that do not harbor the same trigger types is close to impossible in the current health care environment. Today physicians have had to trade practice autonomy for financial security.

One of the ways for physicians to deal with stress triggers at this stage is to tap into another defense mechanism that is easy to deploy, does not carry significant confrontational risk, and is surprisingly "very economic". It is working harder. To a physician in the workaholic stage, working harder offers a magic formula. It helps those who implement it to avoid confrontation at work resulting from one of the three mismatches (moral-economic-intellectual); it has also the benefit of helping to avoid intimacy at home when in the later stages of burnout.

In the above scenario, the main mechanism to avoid negative feelings is to become a workaholic. The other way to avoid the negative feelings produced by a practice-physician misfit is develop a compulsive need to prove oneself. This can lead to working harder and becoming a workaholic. In order to prove self-worth to oneself, the physicians set higher expectations for themselves which can be met only by working harder. This becomes more complex as time passes, and they start to perform many of their practice tasks themselves to meet their own increasingly high expectations. This in turn demands more time to accomplish the work, and a vicious cycle is generated. This is just one example of the "chain reaction" we referred to earlier.

The compulsion to prove oneself is not a conscious plan of action. It is more or less a defense mechanism to maintain self-respect and self-worth in a health care environment that has eroded many of the tools by which physicians have traditionally measured themselves. In other words, this is a pathologic relationship where overworking satisfies the new parameter for measuring self-worth, that is, the "amount" of work equals worth. This is a result of implementing a "working harder defense mechanism" in response to a fractured environment in today's healthcare system. The current working environment is foreign to many physicians and their perceptions of what taking care of patients is all about.

Working harder and enjoying it is a healthy way to work and enjoy life. It delivers pleasure, satisfaction, and sometimes an adrenaline rush. For artists, it produces amazing work that we all enjoy, for academicians it produces excellent research and papers that benefit society, and for physicians it generates great outcomes for very satisfied patients.

Most of us remember the thrill of running a code that led to the survival of a patient. We did not mind what time of day or night the code was called; many of us were high on adrenaline from the rush and excitement of saving a life. This version of "working harder" is a lifestyle choice for some, although it makes them difficult partners to live with. But there is another version of working harder that is pathologic; the one that is practiced by physicians suffering from burnout in an effort to avoid negative feelings and/or feed the compulsive need to prove oneself by the amount of work accomplished.

In my opinion, as we indicated previously, the "Working Harder and The Compulsion to Prove Oneself" stage of burnout is exacerbated by the lack of other mechanisms that were traditionally at the core of the practice of medicine, namely, preserving autonomy and satisfying patient-physician interactions. Therefore, physicians new to a practice, especially those who take over an established physician practice, may be prone to starting down the path of burnout early in their career.

Kaiser-Permanent has implemented a successful program to avoid burnout in a young physician's career. Physicians new to the group practice are protected from a heavy work load for up to 2 years. This is accomplished in two different ways; 1) by limiting the number of patients seen per day allowing for longer and more satisfying physician-patient interaction, and 2) by limiting the total number of patients on a new physician's panel.

This very successful program is not economically possible for a small or medium size practice. Many large organizations do have the economic power to implement such a program, but they do not because they lack the vision of Kaiser-Permanente leadership. These organizations still support a management mentality that categorizes physicians as a commodity rather than as assets.

Doubting Self-Capabilities and Skills

You have always been an excellent physician. You were careful to research things you did not know or were unsure of. Now when you miss something, do not remember the symptoms of a given syndrome, or hear about a new entity, you feel inadequate. You doubt your skills and competencies as a physician. Questions about a peculiar symptom presented by a patient, or specific disease sets are very common in day to day practice. That is why most of us have a subscription to Up To Date. However, when you are suffering from burnout, you perceive these ordinary day to day inquiries as major setbacks, and an indication that your competence is failing. This makes day to day practice even more frustrating and stressful.

This may extend beyond the scope of medical questions and become a behavior of undermining the positive in everything you do. For example, your chief asked you to see a difficult patient for a second opinion. To you, it seems that he asked you to do that because no other physician wanted to deal with the issue and it was "dumped" on you. In reality, your chief and your colleagues think highly about your medical skills. That is the reason why you were chosen to help with a difficult case.

This may progress into a more dangerous pattern of thinking when everything becomes "all or nothing" to you. For example, you like the fact that your chief is assigning second opinions or difficult cases to you, but you become doubtful of your performance when the chief asks another colleague to take care of some of these cases.

To further elaborate on this subject it is best to resort to the concept of "Cognitive Distortion" described in the psychology literature. Cognitive distortion is exaggerated or irrational thought patterns that could perpetuate the symptoms of other conditions like depression and anxiety, which have many inter-exchangeable symptoms and signs with the burnout syndrome.

Wikipedia has an excellent article that summarizes Cognitive distortion into a few paragraphs. They are very relevant and to-the-point and help to supplement the limits of this self-help book.

Here we quote Wikipedia:

"Cognitive distortions are thoughts that cause individuals to perceive reality inaccurately. These thinking patterns often reinforce negative thoughts or emotions. Cognitive distortions tend to interfere with the way a person perceives an event. Because the way a person feels intervenes with how they think, these distorted thoughts can feed negative emotions and lead an individual affected by cognitive distortions towards an overall negative outlook on the world and consequently a depressive or anxious mental state.

Main Types:

The cognitive distortions listed below are categories of automatic thinking, and are to be distinguished from logical fallacies.

I- All-or-nothing thinking (or dichotomous reasoning): seeing things in black or white as opposed to shades of gray; thinking in terms of false dilemmas. Splitting involves using terms like "always", "every" or "never" when this is neither true, nor equivalent to the truth.

Example: When an admired person makes a minor mistake, the admiration is turned into contempt.

II- Overgeneralization: Making hasty generalizations from insufficient experiences and evidence. Making a very broad conclusion based on a single incident or a single piece of evidence. If something bad happens only once, it is expected to happen over and over again.

Example: A person is lonely and often spends most of her time at home. Her friends sometimes ask her to come out for dinner and meet new people. She feels it is useless to try to meet people. No one really could like her.

III- Filtering: focusing entirely on negative elements of a situation, to the exclusion of the positive. Also, the brain's tendency to filter out information which does not conform to already held beliefs.

Example: After receiving comments about a work presentation, a person focuses on the single critical comment and ignores what went well.

IV- Disqualifying the positive: discounting positive events.

Example: Upon receiving congratulation, a person dismisses it out-of-hand, believing it to be undeserved, and automatically interpreting the compliment (at least inwardly) as an attempt at flattery or perhaps as arising out of naïveté.

V-Jumping to conclusions: reaching preliminary conclusions (usually negative) from little (if any) evidence. Two specific subtypes are identified:

1- Mind reading: Inferring a person's possible or probable (usually negative) thoughts from their behavior and nonverbal communication; taking precautions against the worst reasonably suspected case or some other preliminary conclusion, without asking the person.

Example: A student assumes the readers of their paper have already made up their mind concerning its topic, and therefore writing the paper is a pointless exercise.

2- Fortune-telling: predicting negative outcomes of events.

Example: Being convinced of failure before a test, when the student is in fact prepared.

VI- Magnification and minimization: Giving proportionally greater weight to a perceived failure, weakness or threat, or lesser weight to a perceived success, strength or opportunity, so the weight differs from that assigned to the event or thing by others. This is common enough in the normal population to popularize idioms such as "make a mountain out of a molehill". In depressed clients, often the positive characteristics of other people are exaggerated and negative characteristics are understated.

There is one subtype of magnification:

<u>Catastrophizing:</u> Giving greater weight to the worst possible outcome, however unlikely, or experiencing a situation as unbearable or impossible when it is just uncomfortable.

Example: A teenager is too afraid to start driver's training because he believes he would get himself into an accident.

VII- Emotional reasoning: Presuming that negative feelings expose the true nature of things, and experiencing reality as a reflection of emotionally linked thoughts. Thinking something is true, solely based on a feeling.

Example: "I feel (i.e. think that I am) stupid or boring, therefore I must be." Or, feeling that fear of flying in planes means planes are a very dangerous way to travel. Or, concluding that it's hopeless to clean one's house due to being overwhelmed by the prospect of cleaning.

VIII- Should statements: Doing, or expecting others to do, what they morally should or ought to do irrespective of the particular case the person is faced with. This involves conforming strenuously to ethical categorical imperatives which, by definition, "always apply," or to hypothetical imperatives which apply in that general type of case. Albert Ellis termed this "musturbation". Psychotherapist Michael C. Graham describes this as "expecting the world to be different than it is".

Example: After a performance, a concert pianist believes he or she should not have made so many mistakes. Or, while waiting for an appointment, thinking that the service provider should be on time, and feeling bitter and resentful as a result.

IX- Labeling and mislabeling: a more severe type of overgeneralization; attributing a person's actions to their character instead of some accidental attribute. Rather than assuming the behavior to be accidental or extrinsic, the person assigns a label to someone or something that implies the character of that person or thing. Mislabeling involves describing an event with language that has a strong connotation of a person's evaluation of the event.

Example of "labeling": Instead of believing that you made a mistake, you believe that you are a loser, because only a loser would make that kind of mistake. Or, someone who made a bad first impression is a "jerk", in the absence of some more specific cause.

Example of "mislabeling": A woman who places her children in a day care center is "abandoning her children to strangers," because the person who says so highly values the bond between mother and child.

X- Personalization: Attributing personal responsibility, including the resulting praise or blame, for events over which a person has no control.

Example: A mother whose child is struggling in school blames herself entirely for being a bad mother, because she believes that her deficient parenting is responsible. In fact, the real cause may be something else entirely.

XI- Blaming: the opposite of personalization; holding other people responsible for the harm they cause, and especially for their intentional or negligent infliction of emotional distress on us.

Example: a spouse blames their husband or wife entirely for marital problems, instead of looking at his/her own part in the problems.

XII- Fallacy of change: Relying on social control to obtain cooperative actions from another person.

XIII- Always being right: Prioritizing self-interest over the feelings of another person."

Being Overly Concerned with Other's Opinions

We all like to be appreciated and held in high esteem by our colleagues. One of the pathologic versions of this natural need is when the need for approval is constant; it becomes an obsession, and needs to be re-emphasized in every tiny behavior by the people around you. This can fester into a more pathologic form when you find yourself becoming very sensitive to criticism. If a colleague or supervisor calls attention to something that is missed, or could be improved, you immediately interpret it as rejection and disapproval. When suffering from burnout, you may even feel that the chief or colleagues are picking on you specifically.

Ignoring Body Signals and Neglecting Self Needs

This is a common practice for male physicians who are on their way to, or are fully engulfed by Burnout syndrome. The body is sending different signals of distress, warning the physician that lack of sleep and insomnia, missing meals, fatigue, and possibly lower back pain are all early red flags of overwork and extreme stress. These signals are frequently ignored, and overworking is the normal life style now. Occasionally the pain and other symptoms are preserved as "badges of honor" by the inflicted physician.

As the problem progresses, accommodating the need to work harder will be found at the expense of lunch time, dinner time with the family, sleeping, visiting friends, hobbies, or relaxation. The need to work harder to find self-worth results in ignoring one's physical and mental needs and begins to creep into the weekend, gradually consuming the majority of the time that used to be spent outside work.

This process is different from the "overworked physician" who is trying to complete charting during lunch time, or getting to work an hour earlier to get a head start on e-mails and labs. The "overworked physician" is one of the physician-practice mismatch issues that can lead to burnout syndrome. In the "overworked physician" the effort is directed toward completing work, in order to have time for positive activities in their life. They work hard so that they have time for important de-stressors, like family and friends, in an active attempt to balance work and life. Unfortunately, due to the broken nature of the current health care environment, many physicians are unsuccessful in taking advantage of the positive variables in their life.

Revision of Values

How physicians revise their value system so that the exclusive pathologic new parameter, such as completing the job, becomes the new value system is mind blowing to us. Understanding this transition, in our opinion, is critical to further identifying solutions for burnout syndrome and abort it before it becomes a snowball rolling downhill.

In my estimates, the problem is seeded in the manner in which physicians are trained. The value system they use to measure self-respect and self-worth is multi-dimensional. In fact, it hasn't changed much since the days when the Hippocratic Oath was articulated by the Greeks. However, the practice of medicine has changed significantly. And a little history would not hurt here.

Health insurance is a child of the 20th century. We may be able to credit, with a significant degree of confidence, the actions of Baylor Hospital in Texas in the year 1929, as the springboard of health insurance. That was the year that the hospital offered about 1500 teachers a pre-paid plan for their medical care.

It is also very interesting to know that Blue Shield was originally established in 1939 by a collaboration of a few state medical societies, including the ones in California, in an attempt to cover physician services. These were hard times during the Great Depression in the United States. There are questions about the real motive behind creating the pre-paid arrangement of Blue Shield by the Medical Societies. Added to that is the fact that the American Medical Association did not like such an arrangement. They favored an indemnity-based insurance that would reimburse the patient for medical expenses. However, we elected not to address this issue in more depth so as not to digress from the focus of this book.

Suffice it to say that the result of those early forays into health insurance planted the seed of a very controversial variable in today's medical practice: trading practice independence for financial security.

Over time the following insurance creatures were borne: Commercial Insurance, Medicare, and Medicaid. The managed care "child prodigy" was growing fast, as early as the 1960's, as the result of government attempts to contain Medicare expenses. Indeed, the actual history of health care in the 20th century is fascinating. However, the one main theme that we have observed is the failure of managed care arrangements to solve the growing Medicare problem.

The managed care principal was dressed in a different outfit each time it changed, but the arrangement was always the same:

1- Pre-paid amount of premium, by private payer or the government
2- Large group of health providers and hospitals assuming partial or complete risk of financial impact of managing medical conditions
3- Valves that regulate "over usage"

However nice its new wardrobe looked, the changes were cosmetic and continued to fail in patching the holes of the Medicare issue.

What has also happened in the period since the 1960's, is that Medicare has become the leader in dictating guidelines for reimbursement, with private insurances following its lead. It was clear that the system would not be able to support itself in the way it was established, short of increasing the percent of the budget allocated to it in every fiscal cycle.

New formulas that scientifically created reimbursement systems evolved into the resource-based relative value scale (RBRVS) system. It was a "new" valve to control leakage of funds from

Medicare by decreasing physicians' fees.

You may want to consider reading this paragraph from the American Medical Association web site about the history of creating that system:

"In 1992, Medicare significantly changed the way it pays for physicians' services. Instead of basing payments on charges, the federal government established a standardized physician payment schedule based on a resource-based relative value scale (RBRVS). In the RBRVS system, payments for services are determined by the resource costs needed to provide them. The cost of providing each service is divided into three components: physician work, practice expense and professional liability insurance. Payments are calculated by multiplying the combined costs of a service by a conversion factor (a monetary amount that is determined by the Centers for Medicare and Medicaid Services). Payments are also adjusted for geographical differences in resource costs.

The physician work component accounts, on average, for 48 percent of the total relative value for each service. The initial physician work relative values were based on the results of a Harvard University study. The factors used to determine physician work include the time it takes to perform the service; the technical skill and physical effort; the required mental effort and judgment; and stress due to the potential risk to the patient. The physician work relative values are updated each year to account for changes in medical practice. Also, the legislation enacting the RBRVS requires the Centers for Medicare and Medicaid Services (CMS) to review the whole scale at least every five years.

The practice expense component of the RBRVS accounts for an average of 48 percent of the total relative value for each service. Practice expense relative values were based on a formula using average Medicare approved charges from 1991 (the year before the RBRVS was implemented) and the proportion of each specialty's revenues that is attributable to practice expenses. However, in January 1999, CMS began a transition to resource-based practice expense relative values for each CPT code that differs based on the site of service. In 2002, the resource-based practice expenses were fully transitioned.

On January 1, 2000, CMS implemented the resource-based professional liability insurance (PLI) relative value units. The PLI component of the RBRVS accounts for an average of 4 percent of the total relative value for each service. With this implementation and final transition of the resource-based practice expense relative units on January 1, 2002, all components of the RBRVS are resource-based.

Annual updates to the physician work relative values are based on recommendations from a committee involving the AMA and national medical specialty societies. The AMA/Specialty Society RVS Update Committee (RUC) was formed in 1991 to make recommendations to CMS on the relative values to be assigned to new or revised codes in Current Procedural Terminology (CPT®). Nearly 8,000 procedure codes are defined in CPT, and the relative values in the RBRVS were originally developed to correspond to the procedure definitions in CPT. Changes in CPT necessitate annual updates to the RBRVS for the new and revised codes."

My conclusion may sound unacceptable to many of you. I concede that point because we do not know for sure if our conclusions are valid. However, I know that increased study and valid conclusions are absolutely necessary and this is why we invite academicians and researchers to work on the subject of physician burnout more earnestly. To be honest, I will be exuberant if my conclusions are wrong. It will mean that someone has found a better prognosis for the medical profession in the coming 25 years.

I think that trading practice independence for financial security worked as long as the work load was acceptable. But as fees declined, and the work load increased, a major conflict arose between the reality of the finance of medicine and the practice of medicine guided by the Hippocratic Oath. The financial reality versus physician training has given way to an internal conflict in every physician's code of ethics.

This internal conflict causes different physician-status outcomes, as influenced by the positive and negative variables in their personal and work environment. The intensity of the internal conflict also depends upon the individual physician's reserve of positive energy, and his/her ability to recharge this reserve. This positive energy is well known to all physicians. With each patient encounter, depending on its complexity, a transfer of energy occurs between you and the patient, leaving you a bit more depleted every time. Most of us get to the end of the day with nothing left on the inside. This issue of physician energy as it relates to patient encounters creates physician "types". Again, we remind you that the following is solely based on my observation. This information is not meant to persuade you to agree with me, rather it is meant as a road map to guide you as you reflect on your current status. I encourage you to reach your own conclusions.

The Saint Physician

You have met someone like this once or twice over the course of your medical . S/he has endless internal energy with a seemingly bottomless ability to transfer positive energy to others and hardly needs to recharge. Frequently, these physicians are not concerned with financial rewards, even though frequently they are doing very well financially. They have enough internal positive energy left by the end of the day's work that they can carry on with fulfilling personal relationships with their spouses, partners, family, and friends.

Everyone Else

There are different sub-categories when it comes to most of the physicians in the work force. I believe that an individual's level of energy, its sustainability, and ease of recharging is based on the method used to resolve conflict. The way in which a physician balances the conflicting priorities of declining income/increasing work load/trading practice independence for financial security determines the level of their positive energy:

1- Able to resolve the internal conflict by creating ancillary medical services that are not covered by insurance or Medicare, and generating significant cash flow. Minimal need for boosting other positive support systems.

2- Able to resolve the internal conflict by significantly blunting the channels that depletes positive energy exchange during patient encounters, making the work day very mechanical and robotic. However, it saves just enough internal positive energy to have a fulfilling personnel life.

3- Able to resolve the internal conflict by recharging their positive energy frequently during the work day by implementing techniques like relaxation, humor, and colleague interactions throughout their day. This is the category that most of us physicians belong to.

Considering that the burn out rate is reaching 50% in some specialties, especially the ones on the front line such as family practice and emergency medicine, we have speculated the following scenarios:

A- These interventions are not being utilized enough by physicians and this is why this self-help book was born.

B- These interventions are not enough to address the problem and further complementary interventions are necessary by medical societies for larger scale support systems, especially for independent physicians and small to medium size groups.

C- These interventions can work for some physicians with certain characteristics, but overall is not a sufficient solution

D- These interventions when fully implemented, are only as good as frequent oil changes for a car that is constantly in overdrive mode. The oil changes definitely help to keep the car going, but the engine will give up at some point in the future, and much earlier than anticipated. Engines were not designed to work in overdrive mode all the time; neither are physicians.

In summary, a revision of values is necessary to resolve the internal conflicts resulting from external variables that can be partially mediated but not eliminated. A physician can change practice type, practice location, practice associates, practice managers or organizations.

The new value system (the destructive one) has already been laid out and very easy to assimilate: it is the "working harder" value system. The physician has been already working harder but this is the overdrive mode that will lead to burnout. In a pathologic twist of emotions, working harder can temporarily provide a new parameter for deriving some self-fulfillment from practicing medicine, especially when all other parameters have been gradually eliminated.

Working harder is not enough to nourish the need for maintaining self-worth. In the absence of all other parameters that provide for satisfaction and fulfillment from practicing medicine, working harder and longer is not going to do the trick. The problem is that by now a revision of values is a done deal. "Working harder" is the new value system against which the afflicted physician will be measuring and evaluating priorities. It is a downhill course from that point on.

Now I have laid down a few building blocks for you, it is appropriate to refer to the work of the Psychologists "Herbert Freudenberger" and "Gail North". They have theorized that the burnout process can be divided into 12 phases, which are not necessarily followed sequentially.

Please feel free to use these in any order you wish, as a tool to help you explore the current status of your career, and reflect on yourself.

The phases of burnout according to psychologists Freudenberger and North are according as follows:

1- The Compulsion to Prove Oneself:
In the early stages, it starts with higher motivation and voluntarism. This may progress into obsession of proving oneself.

2-Working Harder
When the organization or practice is not the right fit, working harder happens as a result of setting a higher personnel expectations. That may lead individuals to try to do everything themselves to meet their higher expectations. In turn this may require more time to complete the same tasks.

3-Neglecting Their Needs
This may gradually escalate to the point where time devoted to completing work is favored at the expense of friends, family, eating, and sleeping time.

4-Displacement of Conflicts
During this stage there is self awareness that something is wrong, but there is difficulty identifying the etiology. This is when the first physical symptoms may start to manifest themselves.

5-Revision of Values
As completing the job becomes the new value system, emotions start to become blunt. Avoidance and isolationism start to become more of an issue.

6-Denial of Emerging Problems

Which could be as simple as avoiding socialization and being around people, as this may be a source of change in their surrounding. Those employees or professionals do not like to deal with these emerging "problems", leading to social avoidance. Irritability, sarcasm, and more aggression is usually the way they start to be seen by the outside observers.

7-Withdrawal

This stage could be quiet dangerous especially for physicians. This is when alcohol or drugs may be sought as a remedy. Feelings of lack of hope in the current work path or start to emerge.

8-Obvious Behavioral changes that are likely to be noticed by everybody at work

9-Depersonalization and losing the feeling of value in themselves or others.

10-Inner Emptiness that may result in indulging in other activities that can fill the void like overeating, sex, alcohol, or drugs.

11-Depression

12-Burnout Syndrome

Burnout in its full presentation is characterized by decreased mental energy, and is associated with absenteeism, high turnover, and reduced job satisfaction.

Three elements constitute burnout:

(1) Emotional exhaustion

(2) Depersonalization

(3) Low personal accomplishment

Let us dive deeper into each one of these three elements of burnout, as exhibited in the general work force. I would like you to reflect on yourself as a physician and use this as a guide for self-reflection and analysis.

<u>Emotional exhaustion</u>

Are you in a chronic state of physical and emotional depletion as a direct result of continuous stress, either work related or due to increased personal demands?

A great example of a personal demand burn out syndrome that we frequently address in neurology is: Care Giver Burn Out in Alzheimer's disease.

The way emotional exhaustion, regardless of the etiology, manifests itself as both physical fatigue and emotional fatigue, frequently described by employees as: I feel physically and emotionally drained.

<u>Depersonalization and Cynicism</u>

Personalization is a normal process that involves identifying oneself with a group. For example, an officer identifies him or herself as part of a larger officers' group with specific characteristics. This is a normal process.

With depersonalization this identification of oneself with a group becomes pathologic. The affected person identifies themselves more and more with the characteristics of the group by adapting more and more, at the expense of the personal attributes that really make them who they are. They gradually evolve, or "devolve" into becoming a "good example" of this group, but more or less in a mechanical empty way.

For example, as a military officer starts to depersonalize, he or she will see more and more of their personality fading away. Progressively, a more malignant form of the characteristics that emphasize their main existence – as an officer - will emerge, like wearing an immaculate uniform, following rigid orders, being punctual, and having a defined enemy. Adhering to these characteristics becomes almost as important as the real task itself.

Depersonalization may also present itself as cynicism.

Low Personal accomplishment

Performance and productivity plunges as an outcome of exhaustion, cynicism, and depersonalization. Physicians feel that they are much less effective in their job. Job dissatisfaction starts to become a serious issue. Self-doubts about choice and hope in the future of the current career path is now called into question by the burned out physician.

5 MALE VS. FEMALE BURNOUT SYNDROME

Is their a difference between Male and Female physicians when it comes to Burn out syndrome?

In a word, yes.

It is a complex story, replete with differences behind the motivation of each gender to study medicine, an individual's approach to medical practice, gender psychology and lifestyle preferences. The characteristics that make men and women different biologically and psychologically carry over into medical practice. However, one similarity exists, and it is an unfortunate one- both male and female physicians can suffer from burnout syndrome. While the root causes of burnout may differ according to gender, the personal and professional toll that burnout exacts on the physician does not. If not caught in the early stages burnout can be ruinous, and that is what we are trying to prevent here.

To understand how the "cause and effect" of burnout differs between male and female physicians let's examine the following:

the percentages of each gender in today's physician body, gender attributes that affect specialty, the professional and personal challenges that contribute to the onset of the syndrome, and the role that biology plays in all this.

One way to determine the percentages of male and female physicians practicing today is to look at medical school enrollment. We understand that all may not matriculate, but this still remains a fairly good indicator of the gender division in the medical profession. The American Academy of Medical Schools (AAMC) reports that "the total number of men and women applying to and enrolling in medical school is fairly equally split". In the 2013 class, 53% percent of enrollees were male and 47% were female.

Even though enrollment is fairly evenly split, the choice of specialty is not. In general, male and female students choose vastly different directions for their practice, and that choice comes down to psychology. Potential income, lifestyle, and future professional growth are all factors in the newly minted physician's specialty selection, but at the core lie their individual values and their psychology regarding the practice of medicine.

The innate differences of gender psychology cannot be extracted from these decisions. Gender does influence career choices and in this instance, it does demonstrably affect choice of medical specialty.

For example, researchers have found that because women are

psychologically more relationship-oriented than men, they tend to seek specialties that allow for relationships. Gender socialization theory holds that as they are growing up, girls are encouraged to exhibit tenderness, be considerate and kind, and to avoid aggressive behavior. These traditional standards lead women to be much more attuned to relationships. Seeking relationships then leads to seeking a comprehensive care practice, because it relies on forming relationships with the patient, and often with families. This can lead the female medical student to use a specialty of family practice.

Comprehensive care means that the physician wants to consider the patient's psychological state, socialization as it affects health and familial issues as part of the provision of physical health care. These physicians want to provide holistic care, rather than just cardiac care, for example, and so they are frequently involved in caring for the patient, members of the patient's family, and providing social advice, education, and lifestyle support over the span of the patient's life. This takes a more emotional toll on the family physician than say, that of a surgeon who interacts with the patient only pre and post-surgery.

Choosing a specialty that provides the opportunity to develop relationships also means that the physician is going to be less able to disconnect with patients in order to obtain mental and emotional rest. Becoming involved in a patient's life in order to support them as they improve their health, demands emotional involvement on the part of the physician. We would argue that this close relationship with patients holds a direct correlation to physician burnout, as emotional exhaustion created from patient connections builds over the years of practice. Even if a physician wants to leave practice, the emotional tug of "What will happen to my patients?" may cause him or her to stay much longer than they should for their own physical and mental well-being.

Why aren't men more relationship-oriented?

Again, gender socialization theory comes into play saying that boys and men are taught assertiveness as they are growing up. Personal independence is stimulated. They are taught to reject feelings of vulnerability. Gender socialization theory holds that boys and men are taught to be aggressive, non-emotional and goal-oriented, and not to show weakness. Medical school underscores this, teaching physicians (male and female) that any vulnerability is actually weakness. It's no wonder then, that men may be unable to solve or even recognize internal conflicts. If the first internal sign of weakness is detected a man is programmed to shut down rather than process the weakness, understand it and resolve it. It could be argued that if this theory is true, men are set up to experience the depersonalization stage of burnout syndrome from a very young age.

And so, when we circle back to the question of the role that gender plays in burnout syndrome, we see that depersonalization may be the core component that triggers burnout for men, while for women emotional exhaustion due to their affinity for patient relationships may be the trigger for burnout.

Medical students may be learning the pitfalls of family practice early. Statistics show that in the past 15 to 20 years, the number of medical students choosing primary care as a specialty has fallen precipitously. The numbers are falling to the point that observers of the medical profession are worried that we may have a future shortage of primary care physicians. By contrast, medical students are increasingly choosing careers in plastic surgery and emergency medicine. Delivering quality care in these two specialties does not depend upon long term relationships with the patient. It could be argued that in both plastic surgery and emergency medicine the patient is in and out, with no long term relationship necessary for successful patient outcomes.

Whether selected by a majority of male or female physicians, research shows that among General Practitioners (GPs), the prevalence of burnout and other stress related complaints has increased during the last decade. According to BMC Public Health, "The organization of the work of GPs as well as their working conditions (i.e., a high workload, organizational problems) may play a role in the high burnout prevalence among doctors. Several studies among GPs show that work factors such as time pressure, emotional demands, patient factors (e.g., dealing with problem patients), and night calls are important problems associated with ongoing stress" in their work. "Additionally, we know that the conditions of medical work in primary care suggest that physicians are particularly prone to work-family interference and that work-family conflict is an important cause of burnout as well."

A study conducted on this issue by the University of Amsterdam showed that not only is there a gender difference in experiencing burnout, there is also a nationality difference. The study entitled, "Sex differences in physician burnout in the United States and The Netherlands' was published in the Journal of the American Medical Women's Association. Here is what the study found:

"Separate physician surveys were conducted in the United States (n=2326) and the Netherlands (n=1426). Thirty-three percent of US respondents were female (adjusted response rate 52%); 18% of Dutch respondents were female (adjusted response rate 63%). Standardized mean sex differences (effect sizes) in burnout variables were calculated and compared cross-nationally. US women experienced more burnout than US men did (28% v 21%, p<.01), but the sex difference in burnout among Dutch physicians was not significant. Women in both countries worked fewer hours than men did (48 v 56 US, 44 v 56 NL, difference in effect sizes of sex differences between US and NL, p<.001). Although women in both countries described less work control than men, the effect size of the sex difference in the United States was more than twice that in the Netherlands (.34 US v .15 NL, p<.01). Children, home support, and work-home interference were comparable between sexes in the United States. Gender parity in physician burnout in the Netherlands may be due to fewer work hours and greater work control of women compared to those in the United States."

It is startling that "the effect size of the sex difference in the United States was more than twice that in the Netherlands." This would lead one to believe that it is not only the medical profession that has an innate disposition toward the creation of burnout, but that American society at large shares those traits. If that is the case, then are we as Americans primed for burnout by virtue of the fact that we live here, making burnout all the more prevalent once we enter a profession? I am not equipped to answer this, it is just one more thought provoking question raised during the close examination of burnout syndrome.

Not only is there pressure at work, there is pressure in our personal lives as well. Physicians are not just physicians; they are husbands, wives, mothers, fathers, and members of an extended family. These responsibilities bring additional pressure to the physician's day to day life, as does the drama and emotional stress that is part and parcel of most families.

And let's not ignore the physical ramifications of burnout. One study, as reported in the online blog, Healthcare Communications, examined "the association between burnout, depression, anxiety, and inflammation as a risk factor for cardiovascular disease.

Researchers discovered that for women, there was an association between burnout and inflammation (as measured by specific protein biomarkers), but this same association was not found in men. Interestingly, it was depression, and not burnout or anxiety that produced similarly elevated levels of inflammation in men.

The question becomes, what role does a physician's personal life play in burnout syndrome?

Gender plays a role here as well. An article published in Stress and Health reported that "the pattern and strength of significant (burnout) effects differed within the separate analyses of men and women. Work–home conflict was a particularly strong burnout predictor in female physicians, whereas workload was the strongest burnout predictor in male physicians."

Even though the ongoing struggle to balance work and home life seems to contribute more to a female physician's burnout, it appears that both men and women worry about that balance. When PEW Research asked both genders about the level of difficulty in balancing the responsibilities of work and family life, "16% of working mothers and 15% of working fathers say it is very difficult. Overall, 56% of working mothers and 50% of working fathers say it's either very, or somewhat, difficult for them to balance work and family."

The Pew Research survey found that about half (53%) of all working parents with children under age 18 say it is difficult for them to balance the responsibilities of their job with the responsibilities of their family. There is no significant gap in attitudes between mothers and fathers: 56% of mothers and 50% of fathers say juggling work and family life is difficult for them.

The gap that used to exist in the way mothers and fathers spend their time on duties at home and in child care has changed dramatically in the past half century. Dads are doing more housework and child care; moms are doing more paid work outside the home. Neither has overtaken the other in their "traditional" realms, but their roles are converging, according to a Pew Research Center analysis of long-term data on time use.

Despite the fact that roles are converging in the general population, female physicians are suffering burnout that involves the work/life conflict. This would indicate that they feel they are responsible for balancing both. We would make an unscientific assumption that even though they may have a supportive and involved partner; female physicians still feel that they bear the burden of caring for children and organizing the home.

The physician's family is not immune to the effects of burnout, nor are they blind to the physician's struggle to balance work and family. TIME Magazine Medical Insider published an article by Dr. Zachary F. Meisel and Gina Siddiqui called "Can Doctors Have Work-Life Balance? Medical Students Discuss". Here is what one student had to say. His name is Derek Mazique and he is the son of two physicians.

"Both my parents are in primary care, and seeing them practice has been a powerful example of how the field has changed. Perhaps most telling for me is how the current primary care situation is a perfect storm of low reimbursement and doctor burnout. Both of my parents have had to increase the number of patients they see — for my mother who is in private practice, that's the only way she can keep the lights on. I didn't go into medicine in order to emerge as a strictly lifestyle physician … but I did go into medicine expecting to forge meaningful relationships with my patients and to perform my intellectual craft to the utmost. Primary care in its current iteration makes these goals seem even more difficult. Of course, money is a factor, but these expectations of a personally fulfilling medical career also steer my decision-making process."

The decision of whether or not to have children is a burden unto itself, as shown in a body of research conducted in France. The research was developed to discover why the country had difficulty attracting physicians to work in hospitals. One rather stark finding was that 41.3% of female physicians said their profession was an obstacle to having children, compared to 19.3% of the male physicians. The study concluded that "Excessive job demands are linked with burnout and with work-family conflicts, as are difficulties in organizing one's life in order to have and raise children."

So now that we have looked at gender differences, and the different levels of pressure that work/life balance creates for male and female physicians, let's look at how burnout syndrome exhibits itself differently in men and women.

As I discussed earlier, a woman's biological predisposition to involve herself in relationships makes her vulnerable to burnout syndrome in medical practice. The stages with which a female physician experiences burnout stems from her involvement in relationships and then increases from there.

The Female Pattern:

Stage One: Emotional exhaustion

Burnout in female doctors starts with emotional exhaustion. Women traditionally support others in numerous areas of their lives, at home and at work. There is only so much energy and giving to go around. A woman naturally wants to nurture those around her, and this makes it difficult to say no when friends and family need her. Add to that her emotional connection with patients, and emotional exhaustion is a fuse ready to be lit. In Stage One of burnout, a female physician feels that it is becoming impossible to "recharge her batteries", and she begins to blame this on her patients.

Stage Two: Depersonalization and cynicism

This is a dysfunctional coping mechanism. It is a defense

mechanism when a physician feels that their "emotional back" is against the wall. To disconnect and put things at arm's length by feeling cynical about them can make a woman feel better about things for an instant, but it has no long term impact on the feelings of exhaustion. The brain may be saying "I don't care anymore", but the heart is pulling in a different direction toward caring. The dynamic is set in motion and so is the ongoing emotional exhaustion. The female physician increasingly feels "put upon" by her patients, her staff and even the larger health care system. The need to "vent" occurs more often, as does the thought "My patients are trying to drive me crazy." Try as she might, it is difficult for women to maintain cynicism for any length of time. Then comes stage three.

Stage Three: Reduced accomplishment and Self-Doubt

This stage includes a growing doubt about the quality of their practice and the difference that their work makes in their patients' lives. The female physician begins to worry that her work is sub-standard. She cannot recall the motivation for pursuing medicine in the first place. An attitude of "What's the use?" becomes prevalent.

The Male Pattern:

The male pattern of burnout syndrome is different from that of women, and the signs and symptoms exhibit themselves in a different order. For example, whereas women experience depersonalization and cynicism in the second stage, it is the first stage for men.

Stage One: Depersonalization and cynicism

Suddenly, the people who have trained many years to care for are driving you crazy. You need to vent about your patients more often. You can't see why they can't understand what you are talking about. You may even begin to ask yourself why your patients can't take better care of themselves. That is a red flag. It is a response, a dysfunctional one, to the stress of being in medical practice. And it won't help. Venting and complaining will do nothing to deter the efforts of burnout syndrome to slowly cut you down at the knees. While complaining, you will feel badly about complaining, and wonder why you feel a strong need to do so.

Stage Two: Emotional exhaustion

The complaining about patients and venting to colleagues has not helped and emotional exhaustion follows. The male physician is no longer able to cope with the pressures of the practice, and emotional exhaustion sets in until it is nearly debilitating.

Stage Three:

A discussion about burnout was held with Dike Drummond, M.D., a family physician, and posted on HuffPost Healthy Living. It quoted him as describing stage three of burnout for men in the following manner: "By comparison to the female burnout pattern, men's stage three is remarkable for its absence. Male physicians are far less likely to feel that the symptoms of stages one and two affect the quality of the care they offer. This leads to a cynical, exhausted male physician who keeps going despite burnout because he feels he is still a 'good doctor'. The lack of a phase three allows them to continue to practice in denial of their distress, despite the exhaustion and cynicism their coworkers and patients witness on the job."

Although male and female physicians may experience the stages of burnout in a different order, they are more apt to experience the detailed symptoms of each stage in a similar manner. It's important to detail them so that you can detect, as early as possible, if what you are feeling is burnout syndrome.

As Psychology Today reported, the various stages can include any or all of the following symptoms:

Emotional exhaustion stage:

Chronic Fatigue: You lack energy and feel tired often. You may go to bed early, but still wake up tired. You may move more slowly and find you need extra time to get ready and get out the door. At its worse, the fatigue becomes a physical and psychological state of exhaustion. You feel drained. Everything takes a concerted effort. This type of extreme fatigue also often results in a sense of dread for what lies ahead of you on any given day.

Insomnia: In the early stages of burnout, insomnia may be a

problem only one or a few nights each week. Although you feel tired, it may be difficult to fall asleep; or if you do fall asleep, it may be disturbed sleep; or you may wake up in the middle of the night or earlier than you have to. Often, this trouble sleeping relates to persistent thoughts about the insurmountable amount of work that you have to do and whether you'll be able to get it done. In the later stages, insomnia may become a nightly ordeal.

Impaired Concentration and Attention: Physical and mental exhaustion lead to a host of cognitive problems, but the most common are concentration, attention difficulties, and forgetfulness. Because you can't focus, it takes longer to get your work done so things begin to pile up, causing more stress. At its worse, these symptoms prevent you from getting anything done and you simply can't keep up.

Physical Symptoms: All serious physical symptoms, especially chest pains or difficulty breathing, should first be evaluated by a physician to rule out any medical explanations. But it's not uncommon to find that most of the physical symptoms experienced by burnout victims are caused by stress. These symptoms can include chest pains, heart palpitations, dizziness, fainting, tension headaches, migraine headaches, shortness of breath, and stomach pain.

Increased Illness: Because chronic stress depletes and weakens one's body, burnout victims are more vulnerable to infections, colds, flus, and other immune system disorders. The worse the burnout is, the more vulnerable you're likely to be and the longer it's likely to take you to recover from simple infections, like a common cold.

Loss of Appetite: In the early stages of burnout, you may not feel hungry some of the time and may skip meals as a result. In the later stages, this may worsen to a complete loss of appetite and significant weight loss.

Anxiety: Chronic anxiety is common to cases of burnout. Early on, the anxiety may be experienced as nagging feelings of tension, worry, and edginess, which may interfere with your ability to attend and concentrate. Physically, your heart may pound and your muscles may feel tight. Over time, the anxiety may become so severe that it interferes in your ability to go to work or take care of your responsibilities at home. Feelings of apprehension and dread are common. In some cases, the anxiety may become so severe that it results in panic attacks.

Depression:

Although feeling sad from time to time is normal, in cases of burnout, depression is more than just temporary sadness. In the early stages of burnout, you may notice that you're having more bad than good days. It its most severe form, you may feel trapped or think the world would be better off without you. At times, you may become preoccupied with death or dying, or have thoughts of suicide. Obviously, if the depression gets to the point where you're thinking of harming yourself, you should seek immediate professional help.

Anger: Because burnout victims often feel like a failure and experience a lot of guilt, it's not uncommon for these feelings to turn into anger and resentment as the stress continues and you feel as if you have no control over it. At first, the anger may take the form of interpersonal tension with colleagues, family, or friends. As burnout becomes more severe, the anger may intensify and result in angry outbursts and serious arguments at home and in the workplace. You may have thoughts of violence toward coworkers or family, and at its most extreme, this may cross the line into actual violence. When the anger gets to the point where you start thinking of hurting someone else or you cross the line and actually get into a physical altercation, seek professional assistance immediately to prevent anyone from getting hurt, including you.

Depersonalization and cynicism stage:

Loss of Enjoyment: You don't enjoy going to work and then you can't wait to leave. As stress increases, the loss of enjoyment may extend to all areas of your life, including family and friends. At work, you may become preoccupied with thoughts of how you can avoid projects or how you can escape work altogether.

Pessimism: Burnout makes you feel like nothing is going to turn out well. While at one time, you may have been a person who sees the "glass half full," burnout may cause you to feel as if the "glass is half empty," or in some cases, completely empty. This type of negativity is likely to result in feelings of worthlessness, hopelessness, that no one cares or that everyone is out for themselves. This may lead to a lack of trust toward coworkers, family, and friends, increasing tension at home and in the workplace and separating you from social support sources that may once have served as a buffer to your stress.

Isolation: Isolation may start out as mild resistance to socializing, such as not wanting to go to lunch with a coworker or friend. As burnout worsens, you may begin to feel more and more like being alone. Colleagues dropping by to say hello may become an annoyance and you may find yourself closing your door to keep people out. You make excuses not to go out to lunch, or you search for ways to get out of meetings. In the most severe cases, you may get angry at people who approach you. You may even lock your door to keep people away, or come in early or leave late to avoid interactions with colleagues and possibly even family members.

Detachment: In burnout, detachment is a general sense of feeling disconnected to people and your environment. This can take the form of the isolative behaviors described above. In some situations, it may come across as anger toward others. But it also can take the form of detaching yourself emotionally and physically from your job and your responsibilities. For example, you may start calling in sick more often, missing appointments, being chronically late, or not returning calls or emails.

Reduced accomplishment and Self-Doubt

Feelings of Apathy, Helplessness, and Hopelessness: In the beginning, it may seem like nothing is going right. As time goes on, these feelings may become immobilizing, making it seem as if there is no point in getting out of bed.

Increased Irritability: In cases of burnout, irritability is often the result of frustration over feeling ineffective and useless, worsening performance, and a general sense that you're not able to do things like you used to do them. You may snap at people and overreact to minor things. Irritability may create a rift in professional and personal relationships and in the later stages of burnout it may destroy a career, marriages and partnerships.

Lack of Productivity and Poor Performance: Despite long work hours, burnout may prevent you from being able to produce the way you used to, resulting in incomplete projects and work that keeps piling up. It seems like the harder you work, the more ground you lose. You can't climb out from underneath the pile.

Is there a difference in the way male and female physicians ask for help?

There is one gender difference that is a part of every stage of burnout, and that is the willingness to ask for help. Many physicians feel they are alone in practice to begin with. Burnout increases feelings of isolation and keeps feeding itself to prevent the physician from asking for help or support.

It is a classic Catch-22: one of the only ways to recover from burnout is to seek help and yet burnout syndrome tells the sufferer that no one could possibly help.

Remember earlier when I discussed the effect of Gender Socialization Theory on boys and girls as they grow? Boys are taught to be tough, less emotional, and discouraged from acting vulnerable. As men, these teachings serve to dissuade them from seeking help for burnout syndrome. Male physicians may not want to admit even to themselves, that they can't cope or that they aren't tough enough for practice. They will avoid admitting any type of inadequacy or vulnerability. The result is that male physicians hesitate, or avoid, seeking help for burnout syndrome.

Some observers of burnout have noted that men will remain in denial and isolated much longer than women, and that leads to an increased rate of self-medication, relationship failures, addiction, and as statistics show, even suicide.

Women tend to seek help for burnout more than men. Once again the explanation can be found in Gender Socialization Theory. Women seek relationships and that means that they are more likely to have trusted confidantes to whom they feel comfortable admitting that they are emotionally exhausted. Once that information is on the table, close friends can urge the physician to seek help and support.

In the TIME MAGAZINE MEDICAL INSIDER article "Can Doctors Have Work-Life Balance? Medical Students Discuss" Randall S. Bock, M.D., of Revere, Massachusetts discussed the strategies he uses to cope with a busy practice and avoid burnout.

"I have a medical practice with a large component being narcotic-detoxification. I see a large number of addicts whose success rates are not enormous. I run my own medical practice, do the billing, hire staff, see all patients, and deal with whatever consequences occur. I take all of my own night calls, and off-hours I try to keep my family at home intact and happy.

"You need a strong Foundation and your Foundation is strengthened by five F's: Fun, Family, Faith, Friends, and Fur (pets). These F's will help you withstand vagaries in a medical practice.

"Make the most of technology. For instance, I use Dragon dictation, which helps cut down on information-transfer time. Any time you can automate a process and use technology to cut down on the more stultifying aspects of work, consider doing it."

In this same article, Tina B. Tessina, Ph.D., L.M.F.T., from Long Beach, California described her practice experience and the strategies she has developed to avoid burnout. She is a licensed psychotherapist with 30 years' experience in counseling individuals and couples and the author of 13 books in 16 languages. We think her suggestions are great food for thought so as you read them just replace "clients" with "patients" and "therapy" with "medical practice".

She says, "It's necessary to take extremely good care of yourself as the therapist. Here are some specific things to address:

1. Work from your heart – trust yourself and your intuition. If you guess wrong, just accept it and go on. In the end, you have to do therapy your own way. Theories and studies are helpful, but not if they hamper your own style.

2. Identify your preferences, and then do your best to maximize what you like and minimize what you don't like. If you don't like paperwork, get computer programs or secretarial help. If you don't like working with depression, either don't see those clients, or get more training so you'll know how to handle it. If you like working with women, children, couples, etc., focus on that in your practice building.

3. Have a support team of colleagues with whom you can share your therapy experiences as peers.

4. Learn to set solid boundaries. Learn how to say no to intrusive clients, how to keep them in appropriate parts of your life, and not let them take over your free time.

5. Limit your hours to what works for you. Design your own style of working, and make sure your place of work is comfortable to you.

6. Learn from therapists you respect and admire, with whom you feel comfortable. If you don't respect a theory or practice style, don't use it. If you can modify a theory or practice style to suit you, do it."

Resources:

*Medical School Applicants, Enrollment Reach All-time Highs

Gains Increase Urgency to Lift Federal Cap on Residency Training Positions

https://www.aamc.org/newsroom/newsreleases/358410/20131024.html

*Sex differences in physician burnout in the United States and The Netherlands.

http://www.researchgate.net/publication/11059334_Sex_differences_in_physician_burnout_in_the
_United_States_and_The_Netherlands

Department of Medical Psychology, Academic Medical Centre, University of Amsterdam.

Journal of the American Medical Women's Association (1972) 01/2002; 57(4):191-3.

Source: PubMed

*Behrend, T. S., Thompson. L. F., Meade, A. W., Grayson, M. S., & Newton, D. A. (2007, April).
Gender differences in career choice influences. Paper presented at the 22nd Annual Meeting of the
Society for Industrial and Organizational Psychology, New York.

*http://www4.ncsu.edu/~awmeade/Links/Papers/IRT_Med_career(SIOP07).pdf

*Stress and Health, February, 2011. 10.1002/smi.1321

The predictive value of individual factors, work - related factors, and work–home interaction on
burnout in female and male physicians: a longitudinal study

Ellen Melbye Langballe, Siw Tone Innstrand, Olaf Gjerløw Aasland, Erik Falkum

http://www.readcube.com/articles/10.1002%2Fsmi.1321?r3_referer=wol&tracking_action=preview_
click&show_checkout=1&purchase_referrer=onlinelibrary.wiley.com&purchase_site_license=LICE
NSE_DENIED_NO_CUSTOMER

Article first published online: 6 MAY 2010, DOI: 10.1002/smi.1321

Copyright © 2010 John Wiley & Sons, Ltd.

Stress and Health

Volume 27, Issue 1, pages 73–87, February 2011

*MARCH 14, 2013

Modern Parenthood

Roles of Moms and Dads Converge as They Balance Work and Family

BY KIM PARKER AND WENDY WANGhttp://**www.pewsocialtrends.org**/2013/03/14/modern-parenthood-roles-of-moms-and-dads-converge-as-they-balance-work-and-family/

*Work week duration, work-family balance and difficulties encountered by female and male physicians: Results from the French SESMAT study Journal Work: A Journal of Prevention, Assessment and Rehabilitation, Publisher, IOS Press,

ISSN1051-9815 (Print), 1875-9270 (Online)

Issue Volume 40, Supplement 1/ 2011, Pages 83-100

DOI 10.3233/WOR-2011-1270

Online Date Friday, November 18, 2011

*BMC Public Health 2011, 11:240 doi: 10.1186/1471-2458-11-240

The electronic version of this article is the complete one and can be found online at: http://www.biomedcentral.com/1471-2458/11/240

Received: 13 August 2009

Accepted: 18 April 2011

Published: 18 April 2011

*HuffPost Healthy Living Dike Drummond, M.D. Founder TheHappyMD.com

Burnout Presents Differently in Male and Female Doctors

Posted: 08/28/2012 4:44 pm EDT Updated: 10/28/2012 5:12 am EDThttp://www.huffingtonpost.com/dike-drummond/burnout_b_1836998.html

*Burnout Recovery: Stories of Hope

By Janet Scarborough Civitelli, Ph.D. Last updated: Friday, June 14, 2013

http://**www.vocationvillage.com**/burnout-recovery-stories-of-hope/

*CHANGING WORK AND WORK FAMILY CONFLICT

American Sociological Review

2014, Vol. 79(3) 485 –516

© American Sociological Association 2014

DOI: 10.1177/0003122414531435

http://asr.sagepub.com

Published online before print May 4, 2014, doi: 10.1177/0003122414531435

American Sociological Review June 2014 vol. 79 no. 3 485-516

*http://**www.thehappymd.com**/blog/bid/294952/Physician-Burnout-Presents-Differently-in-Male-and-Female-Doctors

*TIME MAGAZINE MEDICAL INSIDER

Can Doctors Have Work-Life Balance? Medical Students Discuss

By Dr. Zachary F. Meisel and Gina Siddiqui Nov. 15, 2011

Dr. Meisel is a practicing emergency physician and assistant professor of emergency medicine at the Perelman School of Medicine at the University of Pennsylvania.

*http://**www.kevinmd.com**/blog Physician suicide 101: Secrets, lies and solutions

*http://**healthcareprcommunications.blogspot.com**/2015/02/women-burn-out-research-roundup-tips-to.html

SOURCE: "The Association Between Burnout, Depression, Anxiety, and Inflammation Biomarkers: C-Reactive Protein and Fibrinogen in Men and Women," [Journal of Occupational Health Psychology: 2005, Vol. 10, No. 4, 344–362], Authors: Sharon Toker and Arie Shirom, Tel Aviv University; Itzhak Shapira and Shlomo Berliner, Tel Aviv Sourasky Medical Center; Samuel Melamed, National Institute of Occupational & Environmental Health and Tel Aviv University]. Full study available at http://www.shirom.org/PDF_new/The_Association_Between_%20Burnout_Depression_Anxiety_and_SharonSJOHP2005.pdf

*Where Do You Fall on the Burnout Continuum?

Recognizing the danger signs of burnout. Post published by Sherrie Bourg Carter Psy.D. on May 06, 2012 in High Octane Women

https://**www.psychologytoday.com**/blog/high-octane-women/201205/where-do-you-fall-the-burnout-continuum

6 THE MANAGER VS. THE CUSTODIAN

A simple shift in mind set can help the manager transition into an effective leader. Managers need to evolve from their typical approach of "managing" assets into "custodians" of their assets. In reality, this is not a very easy task for health care managers because they have to make two significant shifts:

1- Start to think of the physicians they interact with as assets rather than commodities
2- Start to think of themselves as custodians of assets rather than managers of assets.

What does it take to successfully undertake this seemingly simple shift in mind set?

First, it takes the right person; someone who is a leader, not a number cruncher. A "custodian" manager feels a personal responsibility to his or her staff and derives significant pride from keeping staff members in their most intact, polished form. When it comes to treating physicians as assets, the custodian is motivated to find solutions to help them perform at their best and highest level while at the same time protecting them in their best shape - shiny, polished, and intact. The "custodian" manager feels that staff has been entrusted to them and that it is his/her responsibility to care for them.

What are the differences between the characteristics of an effective leader and those of a lower level manager?

1- Proactive, while a manager is usually reactive

2- A leader is enthusiastic and charismatic, while a manager is usually predictable and does not have the infectious energy of a leader.

3- Open minded in adjusting goals and objectives to meet business challenges, while a manager is excellent in carrying out the mission that has been delegated down the management hierarchy.

4- A leader is a delegator

    a. Able to create a team of competent people that can enable effective delegating

    b. A manager is an implementer, carrying out directives.

5- Open to change from the bottom up, as much as changes from the top down. A manager often does not have enough power to effect change.

6- A good listener

7- Flexible

8- Dedicated. A high level of dedication can expose these leaders to burnout syndrome; just like the assets they are trying to protect- the physicians.

9- Leaders are creative and resourceful, even with the limited means they may have. They are able to create solutions in their own locale because they are able to successfully connect with people, motivate them, lead them, and achieve results through commitment and dedication. A manager is not given the latitude to conduct themselves in this way. They are tasked with managing, not creating.

Managing Physicians vs. Managing Practice

A simple shift in mind set can help a manager become a leader. It involves an evolution from their typical approach of "managing" their practice, to becoming the "facilitators" in their practice.

As a manager, the approach to practice management should be like steering a moving ship; one is focused on not making any large-scale, abrupt changes that can shake the balance of passengers and goods. Instead, changes are always minute and smooth, the best route has already been charted and the destination is clear. If planning is done correctly, major decisions are not made frequently and on the fly, rather they are made strategically. A good manager makes decisions once s/he has taken into consideration multiple mitigating factors, the impact on staff, and any other issues that will affect the outcome.

The physician mind set is very different from that of the typical effective manager. A physician is trained to think dynamically and to quickly make major life and death decisions multiple times a day. Physicians are trained to, and capable of, functioning with complete autonomy. They make their patient care decisions "now", not after gaining wide consensus.

For a manager, this approach is very difficult to accept and understand. Managers may consider it as "shooting from the hip". In private, managers tend to think that physicians (male and female) are a "bunch of cowboys" and that trying to manage them is tantamount to "herding cats". This lack of understanding of physician training and temperament can result in the imposition of policies that restrict physician behavior, not necessarily to the benefit of the organization. In an effort to root out what managers may consider impulsive behavior, they create an environment in which physicians feel pressured and constrained. This may in turn adversely affect their ability to practice medicine to their highest and best ability.

On the other hand, when a leader, rather than a manager, solves this problem, there is a completely different solution. The leader focuses on facilitating the physicians' ability to function comfortably and with autonomy. The leader understands the physician's inherit ability to make decisions "now" and capitalizes on that by ensuring that they are well-informed about hospital operations. This is the leader's ability to share the steering of the ship with physicians, suggesting fine adjustments that will facilitate the steady steering of the ship through the rough seas (organizational challenges) that may lie ahead. This approach is in stark contrast to managers who try to supervise physicians with the mantra "the less they know the easier it is to manage them".

Kaiser-Permanente has done a very good job of keeping their physicians informed of the ship's progress. Changes and news about the organization are communicated on multiple levels. First, management meets with the leaders of a small, local group of 10 to 12 physicians. They meet on a weekly or bi-weekly basis. Then the meetings are expanded and communication sessions are held regularly, but less frequently, at local and regional facilities.

The organization also has a handle on how to develop physician leaders. The most important point is that they are handpicked to participate in the leadership development program. A refining process takes place over the course of 7 to 10 years that identifies and develops these candidates for leadership. It starts in the first 2 years of a physician joining the group. This is the time period when physicians are identified as having leadership potential, based on input from physician colleagues and medical chiefs. In the ensuing years the physicians' skills are sharpened through leadership courses. Their development is tested and refined constantly by participation in different leadership tasks ranging from the simple to the complex. This sophisticated system is almost guaranteed to consistently produce the excellent leadership talent necessary to govern Kaiser-Permanente.

Authority vs. Collaboration

The dominant styles of leadership are defined as authoritative and collaborative. Here we summarize the basic differences between the two modalities:

Authoritative based leadership	Collaborative based leadership
1- Power comes from authority	1- Power maximized by team collaboration
2- Maintain ownership of information	2- Openly share information and knowledge
3- Feedback welcome though appropriate channels	3- Feedback is critical to successful leadership
4- Solutions are a product of the board room	4- Solutions are product of brain storming

A. Authoritative leaders are heavy-handed in utilizing their powers. As a result, they can undermine their own ability to develop relationships. They also dampen creativity and innovation in their corporations.

B. Conversely, when collaborative leaders go too far in their enthusiasm about their leadership principals, they can slip into a "popularity trap".

C. We believe that the authoritative leader is the same as a manager, in that they direct rather than lead, while the collaborative leader is more or less a politician.

In my opinion the most successful leadership style for current health care organizations is a "flexible arrangement" style, that is; the core of the management style should be collaborative while exercising authoritative behavior. Exercising authoritative behaviors within a collaborative leadership style will protect the leader from slipping into a popularity trap, and it will provide a daily reminder that the ship has a captain.

A recent article in the Healthcare Press addressed the collaborative leader: "The entire healthcare industry is undergoing revisions to its philosophy with a newfound focus on collaboration. The emphasis on cooperative attitudes means a CEO's ability to work out of hierarchal bounds — and abandon a divide-and-conquer mindset — is crucial to the hospital's success. This ability is partially generational but also something people can develop professionally. "I think some of this change is the most difficult for traditionally-trained leaders to adapt to," says Kim Smith, a former hospital CEO and current partner with executive search firm Witt/Kieffer, who has seen this firsthand. Ms. Smith. "It's not about who owns the power anymore. It's about managing the relationship."

Of course this is my contribution to the subject and may contradict today's mainstream writings and popular musings on leadership. But again, I remind you that if current leadership styles were successful in supporting physicians, burnout rates would be lower in health care organizations. As we have discussed in other chapters, physicians who have supportive management are less likely to suffer from burn out.

It is Time for CEOs to Understand What Physicians Do

For this paragraph I elected not to write any of my own thoughts, but instead to insert this paragraph, word for word. This is the introduction to an article written by "Uwe Einhardt" on January 10, 2015 and published online in "Modern Healthcare". The article is entitled, "Commentary: Why hospitals need a different physician management model".

"If I believed in reincarnation, I would think that American hospital CEOs must have done something wicked in an earlier life to be condemned to their current role in this life.
After all, what other managers in modern economies are asked to manage enterprises over whose costs they have so little control? The bulk of their costs are incurred over the signatures of independent, itinerant professionals—self-employed physicians, who view the hospital as their free workshop whose employees they can order to do this or that, incurring this or that cost for the

hospital—all without taking any responsibility for the costs they have triggered with their orders. On top of all that, they get privileged parking, free of charge! Could this work in any other branch of the economy? Surely not."

Who is Uwe Reinhardt"? According to "Modern Healthcare"; Uwe Reinhardt is the James Madison professor of political economy at Princeton University. He is currently a director of Boston Scientific Corp., a medical-device company, and a trustee for the Hambrecht & Quist Life Sciences Fund and Health Care Fund, which are closed-end mutual funds.

Top CEOs are Physicians

This statement is true, according to a paper written by Amanda H. Goodall and published in "Social Science & Medicine" entitled, "Physician-leaders and hospital performance: Is there an association?"

The authors of the paper collected data on the top 100 U.S. hospitals, as ranked by US News and World Report in 2009, in three specialties: cancer, digestive disorders, cardiac and cardiac surgery. The personal histories of 300 chief executive officers within these hospitals were traced and divided into physician and non-physician manager classifications.

The study found a strong positive association between the ranked quality of a hospital and whether or not the CEO was a physician. The author concludes at the end of the abstract: "This kind of cross-sectional evidence does not establish that physician-leaders outperform professional managers, but it is consistent with such claims and suggests that this area is now an important one for systematic future research."

I have discussed these findings in another chapter, but I consider this evidence to be worth repeating.

How do Successful CEOs Think?

In today's dynamic and sometimes chaotic healthcare environment, successful CEOs are fast on their feet and innovative in addressing challenges, while remaining cognizant of the traditions ensconced in the field of health care. They are willing to learn from competitors, and base important decisions on best practices in the industry.

A successful CEO listens to people cleaning the floor just as intently as they listen to the Chief Medical Officer. They seek input from employees at all levels, communicate consistently, and foster collaboration and communication. In other words, a successful CEO is not myopic, rigid nor isolated.

These traits are at the core of good leadership, and exist in hospitals where the physicians are treated as assets rather than commodities.

How do Successful CFOs Think?

CFOs are a different type of executive. They live by financial rules and regulations. Their world is black and white and ruled by the spreadsheets that tell them how they are performing. It can be said that Chief Financial Officers are not collaborative by nature, rather they are logical, methodical and directed by hard numbers that do not lie. Chief Financial Officers carry the responsibility of building, maintaining and protecting the positive financial performance of the organization. Therefore, all decisions are made in that light, including decisions regarding physicians and their practices.

A successful CFO has financial foresight, a deep understanding of the business, the ability to set goals that are measurable and achievable, and the confidence to make decisions that may involve calculated risk.

How to shift from being a successful CFO to a successful CEO

The transition from CFO to CEO can only be successful when the CFO is no longer viewed as a mere functional specialist, but as one of a company's future leaders. Statistics show that this transition happens frequently in large corporations.

A Financial Executive survey conducted in 2000 of companies with revenues greater than $500 million, revealed that 33 percent of responding CEOs had risen through the finance ranks, while only 26 percent had reached the top from operations and 21 percent from sales and marketing. A survey of Fortune 1,000 CEOs by the executive search firm Heidrick & Struggles found that 36 percent of CEOs were grooming their CFOs for a general management position, and 33 percent were usually considered CEO candidates. In turn, most of the Fortune 1,000 CFOs (72 percent of those surveyed) were grooming a successor to take over the finance function in anticipation of their own advancement.

The results of CFOs becoming CEOs are mixed. Some transitions end in disaster while others are successful in building stable, profitable companies. One man who successfully made the transition from CFO to CEO is John Dasburg, CEO of Burger King. Dasburg was the CFO of Marriott International Inc. during a period of enormous change and growth in the 1980s, when much of its value creation came from a complete restructuring of the way it developed and managed its properties. He was also CEO of Northwest Airlines through its very rocky 1990s, which included rancorous labor negotiations, a barely averted bankruptcy filing and, in 1999, a late-night call from a plane full of irate, stranded passengers on a snow-covered Detroit runway. Having been through periods of enormous change in both positions, Dasburg is quite clear on the different demands of the two jobs.

"When you move from being a CFO to being a CEO, you have to change the way you think, act and communicate," he said recently. "A CEO must think at a higher level of abstraction – more inductively and less deductively. A CEO must be more willing and able to act on key decisions with fewer facts, relying more on grounded assumptions. And a CEO must be able to communicate effectively to a broader constituency – in particular, he must be far more politically attuned."

Pitfalls of CFOs when they become CEOs

I think it is best said by a report in the online edition of Financial Executive:

"What is most surprising is that when a CFO moves into the company's CEO position, they often find themselves unprepared to deal with an altogether different set of challenges - having less to do with financial know-how and more to do with the intangibles of leadership," says Thomas Neff, U.S. Chairman of executive search firm Spencer Stuart, who has placed many executives into CFO and CEO positions. "CFOs who are successful as CEOs have often ventured well outside their traditional financial oversight role and learned all aspects of the business - from building a relationship with the board to line management."

How does a CFO adapt to become a successful CEO?

First and most importantly, to become a successful leader in the CEO chair, a CFO must change their mind set and the way in which they approach problem solving. It is not easy to change a lifetime of training and approach to business challenges, but a CEO must think in a very different way from a CFO. Let's look at the CEO thought process that the CFO must adapt.

Collaborative, fast paced decision making

The CFO, as a newly appointed CEO, must apply his or her skills in a much faster-paced – and less controlled – context. A study conducted almost 30 years ago by management theorist Henry Mintzberg found that the median time spent by a CEO on any one issue was less than nine minutes. Imagine how that time has been shortened in today's digital, connected world. CEOs have to gather facts, consult colleagues, make assumptions, consider alternatives, make decisions and move on to the next issue in a disciplined and sometimes ruthless way.

Accountability and Results

The second distinctive characteristic of the CEO job is the fact that, as Harry Truman liked to say, "The buck stops here." CEOs are accountable for action and results, more so than any other position in the company. At the same time, because of the complexity and urgency of their decisions, they are least likely to be able to predict outcomes. It is rare that any decision having a major impact on a company – strategy shift or a reorganization – can be made with full knowledge of its likelihood of success.

Motivation

The third skills challenge for the CFO-turned-CEO is in the area of motivation. It's not that CFOs don't need to motivate, but that for CEOs, it's a bigger part of the job. CEOs must be able, through strong leadership, to build consensus across a broad set of constituencies.

Practically speaking, how does a CFO train to become a great CEO?

What elements are key to transitioning from a tactician to a successful leader?

Most of the literature on becoming a CEO, whether you are coming from a CFO position or another specialty, reports that the path to the CEOs office begins early in one's career. A successful CEO has experience in many different areas of the company. They have worked in operations, finance, sales and marketing. They have worked on the floor, on the front lines, in emergency rooms, policy, and government. They have headed local and regional divisions. In other words, they know the details of how the company is run and what makes it tick. Their experience in different facets of the industry gives them a holistic view when making decisions that affect the company. When a CFO transitions into the CEO chair, s/he must learn to think, act, work, relate, communicate and make decisions with a broader perspective than when based in finance.

If you want to be a CEO, you must consider the following strategies. In the book, "How to Become CEO, The Rules for Rising to the Top of Any Organization", author Jeffrey J. Fox details the fine tasks that must be studied and adopted by those wanting to become a CEO. I reprint them here with a nod to Jeffrey for his comprehensive list, and we have added some of our own notes regarding practicing these tips in a health care environment:

1. Don't Expect the Personnel Department to Plan Your Career - Human Resource departments do not have a grand plan for you. Your career growth is your responsibility, and no one else's.

2. Keep Physically Fit - Ninety percent of all people climbing the corporate ladder are out of shape. Being fit will give you the energy and motivation to succeed. *After all, you are leading a health care organization. You are the face and voice of the hospital now. How can you talk about wellness if you are not well?*

3. Do Something Hard and Lonely - Do something that you know very few other people are willing to do. All great and

successful athletes remember the endless hours of seemingly unrewarded toil. So do CEOs. *Plan to spend a holiday with the on duty staff instead of at home. It is an extraordinary gesture to show them their value and their worth to the institution. It will also show you as a leader that considers staff an asset instead of a commodity.*

4. Never Write a Nasty Memo - It's unprofessional, regardless of the circumstances. Plus, the world of business is very small; it could come back to bite you in any number of ways. Spend your energy on positive things. *Written notes never go away. Somewhere, someone has them. Your words, taken out of context, will be your undoing. If you have mentioned names, you are in big political trouble. Health care has the memory of an elephant anyway. You don't need to provide written evidence to help the gossip along.*

5. Think for One Hour Everyday - Plan, dream, scheme, think, recharge, calculate. Figure out how to get things done. Take mental stock. Do this every day. *You may wonder where, when or how you are supposed to do this. Changes in health care are coming in like a Tsunami. An executive that does not take time to reflect can quickly become out of touch and swept away by minutia.*

6. Know Everybody by Their First Name - To most people, there is no sound sweeter than their name remembered and pronounced correctly. People will appreciate it. *As leader*

of a health care organization, you need to walk through your facility every week, if not every day. You need to know the nurses, as well as the doctors. You need to know the volunteers, and the people at the registration desk. No one wants to be an anonymous face in the crowd to their employer. When you know a person's name, when you acknowledge a job well done, you have empowered that employee to do more, go farther and work harder.

7. Make One More Call - The difference between the successful person and the average is inches. The person who goes the extra step or two every day is going to be the best.

8. Send Handwritten Notes - They stand out. They are personal, and never out of style. Send one handwritten note a week...for starters. *We have witnessed this personally- a CEO spending hours each week writing handwritten thank you notes and notes of recognition to front line employees. We heard stories of them showing their families and proudly posting on their refrigerator at home. When a simple act builds loyalty for the cost of a stamp- that is enormous ROI for the organization.*

9. Don't Hide an Elephant - The longer you hide a big problem the more you increase its severity. If possible, turn a big problem into an opportunity to shine. *Don't think that because you don't talk about a problem, no one knows about it. Hospitals are notorious for having high developed*

"grapevines". If you don't tell the employees, someone else will. The worst thing that can happen is that if you don't tell the employees first, they will read it in the news. Be transparent, be honest, and trust your employees. They can handle the bad news as well as the good. They may have good ideas for solutions and even rally to help. Physicians are the same. Rather than create increased pressure with silence over the financial situation of the hospital, be honest, let them step up to help.

10. Always Say "Yes" to a Senior Executive Request - Always say "I can do it" when a top manager asks. Then, give him or her more than s/he asked for, and sooner than expected. People who get the job done are the ones who get the top jobs. *As an executive, consider internal recognition programs. Health care is the home for committed, passionate professionals. Nurses will sleep at the hospital so a young mother doesn't have to drive through a snowstorm to get to work. Physicians will stay by a patient's bedside or support a colleague just because it is the right thing to do. Thank them publicly. It's what a good leader does.*

11. Over invest in People - Hire the best people. Attract, motivate, train, and reward the best people. Leaders know that people make things happen. Hire people according to the three "I's": "I" for integrity, "I" for the "I can do it" attitude, and "I" for intelligence.

12. "Stop, Look, and Listen" - CEOs reflect, think, consider, ponder, observe, probe, and listen. Train yourself to always be on "high receive." Good listeners are considered great conversationalists. Listening is equated with wisdom and intelligence.

13. Homework, Homework, Homework - Many people in business never really work hard. But there is a lot of activity, often busywork. This is the "rocking chair syndrome" - lots of movement, but they're not going anywhere. Hard workers do the hard things and they do their homework. Success in projects is anticlimactic. Homework preordains it.

14. Treat All People as Special - Excellent managers make people feel that they are: asked, not questioned; overpaid, not underpaid; measured, not monitored; people, not personnel; sold on what to do, not told; instrumental, not instruments; workers, not worked; contributors, not costs; needed, not heeded.

15. Be a Credit Giver, Not a Credit Taker - Give everybody 100% credit for the work they do. Many managers feel that if their people look too good, they'll be diminished. The credit taker is insecure, dishonest, and known to all. Give proper credit and you will get your due.

I think that Jeffrey Fox has it right.

CEOs; The Good and The Bad

I think there is honor in being very good at your job as CEO at a local or regional hospital. When you are the CEO of a multi-national corporation, your leadership style becomes known on a much larger stage, for better or for worse. The world knows about your positive contributions or misdeeds. There is a lot to be learned from the actions of both. I would like to add that even though neither of the following examples are from health care, leadership is leadership, and the traits of these two CEOs would either build or destroy any organization they led.

Entrepreneur magazine printed profiles of two CEOs, Indra Nooyi.

Chairman and CEO of PepsiCo as an example of world-caliber leadership and Dick Fuld, former chairman and CEO of Lehman Brothers as an example of world-caliber greed and unethical practice. Only one served as CFO on her way to CEO.

Nooyi started at PepsiCo in 1994 as chief strategist. She later served as senior vice president, CFO and president. She was named CEO in 2006 and chairman in 2007. PepsiCo employees approximately 300,000 employees worldwide and has an annual revenue of $60 billion.

As a leader at PepsiCo, Nooyi helped spin off Pepsi's restaurant division in 1997, restructuring KFC, Pizza Hut and Taco Bell into a separate company, Yum Brands. In 1998 she put together a $3.3

billion deal for the purchase of Tropicana, and was instrumental in deciding to sell Pepsi's bottling operations (valued at $2.3 billion in its 1999 IPO). In 2000, Nooyi helped make one of the biggest food deals in corporate history when Pepsi acquired Quaker Oats for $13.4 billion. She was also instrumental in beating out archrival Coca-Cola for beverage-maker SoBe, which Pepsi acquired for $337 million. Since Nooyi was named CFO in 2000, Pepsi's annual revenue has risen 72 percent. Net profit from 2000 to 2006 more than doubled to $5.6 billion.

When asked how she would describe her leadership style, Nooyi said she strategizes 24/7: "I wake up in the middle of the night and write different versions of PepsiCo on a sheet of paper." She also strongly promotes Pepsi's diversity and inclusion training and leadership programs for employees--and studies teamwork by watching replays of Chicago Bulls championship games.

Former Pepsi CEO Steven Reinemund has called Nooyi "a deeply caring person" who "can relate to people from the boardroom to the front line." We call your attention to the fact that it is no accident that she relates to people at all levels of the organization, something that we have referred to repeatedly as one of the traits of an effective leader. Nooyi says "If you want to improve the organization, you have to improve yourself, and the organization gets pulled up with you."

At the absolute opposite end of the leadership spectrum is Dick

Fuld, former chairman and CEO of Lehman Brothers. He started at Lehman in 1966 as an intern and was hired in 1969 as a commercial-paper trader. He held the CEO and chairman position from 1994 until 2008, when the firm filed for Chapter 11 and announced a sale of major operations to parties that included Barclays Bank. The company employs more than 25,000 employees, with $4.2 billion in net income on net revenue of $19.3 billion in 2007. After filing for bankruptcy with $639 billion in assets and $619 billion in debt, Lehman saw its market share fall by more than $46 billion.

It is widely considered that Fuld steered Lehman into bankruptcy. He has been criticized for not completing, or refusing, several proposed deals that may have kept the firm afloat, and for underestimating the effect of the U.S. housing market's collapse on Lehman's mortgage bond underwriting. His board of directors was known to be slow or reluctant to challenge him on his decisions as share prices fell. In the 2 years before the firm's collapse, Fuld's take-home pay was $40.5 million in 2006 and $34 million in 2007.

He was nicknamed the "Gorilla of Wall Street," reportedly for his combative personality and tendency to grunt. In the Wharton School of Business' online journal, Fuld offered the following leadership advice: Pick a strategy and stick with it, "unless of course, you're wrong." He ruled with an iron fist and bankrupted the company.

That brings us to the concept of team work.

Are you only as good as the people that you surround yourself with? Is that of any consequence in health care leadership? I would answer both of those questions with a resounding yes.

A team is defined as an interdependent group of employees who unite around a particular task or objective. It is also a group that supports the CEO and can help to implement initiatives and build a positive corporate culture. A team approach to the work can result in an organization treating physicians like assets, rather than commodities.

Richard Cordova just stepped into the role of chairman of the American College of Healthcare Executives and recently addressed the 2015 Congress on Healthcare Leadership in Chicago. In his address Cordova said that you are only as good as your team: "Admitting your weaknesses takes courage, but in doing so you can surround yourself with people who complete you," Mr. Cordova says. "I'm fond of saying that I'm a mile wide and an inch deep on issues. So I hire people who are a mile deep and an inch wide on those issues."

To discover what our future leaders are thinking about teamwork, we referred once more to Entrepreneur magazine, where in a recent article contributor Marty Fukuda, Chief Operating Officer of N2 Publishing talked about the importance of teamwork:

"Achieving success in business requires the support of mentors, cheerleaders, coaches and partners. A lifetime of victories, however, is rooted in the inspirational backing of a team. To find yourself with dependable backers, you must be willing to return the favor, remain humble and share your success.

Here are five quick tips to keep in mind as you look to build a winning team.

1. Treat people right.

You learned it in kindergarten -- treat others how you want to be treated. When you go out of your way to help others, you can usually expect the same in return. Not to mention it feels great knowing you've contributed to someone else's success.

2. Shun arrogance.

Arrogance is unattractive no matter what your achievements. If you present yourself as though you're already the best, how could anyone, including your supporters, ever help you? A humble professional, however, never lacks support, new opportunities and promising chances.

3. Have a motive greater than yourself.

If you treat others with respect and avoid the pitfalls of arrogance, you will likely gain support -- but why stop there? If your motivation isn't simply personal gain but achieving success for a larger, greater good, support can grow into fanaticism. In this beautiful way, fans will rally for the larger purpose, inspiring and uplifting all involved.

4. Give credit where credit is due. (This isn't the first time we have seen this advice!)

If you surround yourself with the right people, they'll take pleasure in helping you. In return, show your appreciation by helping others. Thank employees, staff and colleagues publicly, privately and often for their important contributions.

5. Collaborate. (There it is- the importance of collaboration.)

A great team beats a great individual any day. When you surround yourself with other like-minded folks with a winning mind set, you benefit from fresh ideas, profound insight and good energy."

Teamwork is part of the greater good

In a healthcare setting, teamwork is becoming a best practice. Consider the teams that care for complex patients, or the teaching sessions that take place in 15 minutes on the nursing floor. A physician visits for a quick "teaching in the round" so bring nursing up to date on a specific skill or patient care issue. When teamwork is combined with best practices and strong leadership, you have a recipe for a strong healthcare organization that can optimize patient care and safety.

The Agency for Healthcare Research and Quality (AHRQ) was one of the first to study the role of teamwork in preventing hospital-acquired patient infections. The study addressed central line infections that occurred in intensive care units, infections that can be deadly to the patient. "By following this teamwork-based approach, hospitals prevented more than 2,000 infections, saved 500 lives, and avoided more than $34 million in health care costs."

So if teamwork is powerful enough to save lives, imagine what it can do to motivate employees; imagine what it can do to take advantage of the skills and talents of physicians in the organization, to treat them as team assets, rather than corporate commodities.

Resources:

Amanda H. Goodall that was published in "Social Science & Medicine" Volume 73, Issue 4, August 2011, Pages 535–539 by "" and titled: Physician-leaders and hospital performance: Is there an association?

Making the Leap from CFO to CEO By Paul Favaro http://**www.favaro.net/**publications/cfo-to-ceo/CFOtoCEO.htm

http://www.**entrepreneur**.com/article/222799

7 THE BAD MANAGER

The bad manager is not an evil person on a mission to harm physicians and turn their professional and personnel life into hell. A bad manager, when it comes to physicians, is usually a trained professional who is superb in mining data, dealing with numbers, and has very good people skills, but no insight into the managing of physicians. So the end result is that bad managers can frequently, albeit sometimes unintentionally, harm physicians and turn their professional and personnel life into hell.

In order to get to know this manager better, I am going to walk you through several concepts. You can form your own opinion about which may be the characteristics of a bad manager that you know. All bad manager are bad, but not in the same way.

Concept #1: A manager is someone who carries out a corporate policy

A manager, no matter what the accompanying title or rank, is someone who is trusted to carry out the policies of the corporation or organization and ensure that said policies are implemented according to set guidelines.

A manager's performance is monitored by superiors, and long term job security and advancements depend on the ability to continue to deliver on the corporate mission. The manager can be only your "friend" or "buddy" as long as your goals are aligned with his/hers and your path parallels the manager's.

In general, managers have to be good tacticians who can see to it that the dictated down strategies can be delivered successfully. They are excellent in execution, but not in innovation.

So what do these managers think of physicians in general?

They don't understand them.

Executives and physicians have different training, different motivations for the work, and a different thought process about business. Executives really don't understand physicians. For the most part, physicians don't understand business, and don't want to. They want to practice medicine. The diverse training of executives and physicians makes it difficult for them to see eye-to-eye, even as new healthcare policies are making the integration of the two essential, if not required.

Physicians are by nature, independent, autonomous, and driven by evidence-based procedure. Speculation is not part of a physician's training. Physicians are also entrepreneurial; they have to be to establish an independent practice, especially one that can survive in the current highly regulated healthcare environment.

John Hsu, MD posted a comment in response to an online article in Becker's Hospital Review regarding the issue of physician/executive integration. We think it is an articulate summary of physician frustration with the business of healthcare.

"Unhappy physicians tend to be associated with more errors of either omission or systems issues. Ironic that the goal of improving the quality of care has the opposite effect. I believe it is because the regulators of medicine have treated the symptoms or problems of our healthcare system ills rather than the cause. How can we fix it? Unfortunately it will be in the form of a single payor. Sure we physicians are poor performers in business but at least when the ACA - ObamaCare determines that our fees will by 30% but will make up the difference by giving us more patients, I perceive the reality that I will essentially only see the 30% cut. I am already working at my maximum. I work 60-80 hours a week already. Make me work harder and I will begin to take shortcuts and I will begin to make errors. It is human nature and it is inevitable. That is why I will retire soon and put in an application at Costco."

Executives are frustrated with physicians because they want to run practices in the same way in which they run the hospital, and that rarely works. Executives don't understand several key characteristics of physicians and their practices:

1. The extent to which physicians are independent-minded and how this impacts communication and decision making;

2. A hospital can't just absorb a physician practice into the organization and run it like the hospital without impacting practice revenue

3. Executives don't understand why they can't integrate physician practice technology into the hospital technology immediately.

To the executive this all makes perfect sense and it is a stretch for them to understand the physician's point of view. Moreover, the executive may have a lack of respect for the physician who is considered a commodity, rather than an asset.

The article that appeared in Becker's Hospital Review and reference above, provides important insight into the executive/physician dichotomy. We quote excerpts here:

"The following are three aspects of integration that hospital CEOs and other executives tend not to understand:

1. Physicians crave input. Hospital administrators and physicians, though they both work in healthcare, were not trained in the same way. Many physicians are entrepreneurial and independent-minded, and they have learned throughout their education to be accountable for their own actions. Many times, however, hospital administrators fail to take this into account and physicians feel they

are a commodity.

2. Physician practices aren't hospital departments. For instance, billing processes are different for hospitals and physician practices and shouldn't be done in the same way. Another similar problem arises with ancillary services. Hospital executives generally want to integrate with a successful — profitable — physician group. But when hospitals acquire and integrate physician groups, they tend to take the ancillary services to the hospital setting — but those ancillary services are usually the very thing that made the practice profitable.

3. Switching technology isn't easy. A large component of hospital-physician integration is technical integration, and hospital executives focus on moving new physician groups onto one system quickly after a deal is made.

That disruption will negatively affect physician morale and productivity and can strain relationships."

Concept # 2 the Extreme CEO

This concept is self-explanatory through this story from Orange County, California published on "The Advisory Board Company", and we quote:

Jury: Health system CEO framed physician by planting gun

CEO wanted to 'humble' dissenting doctor, attorney says

February 14, 2013

A jury has ordered a California hospital chain to pay physician Michael Fitzgibbons $5.7 million after its former CEO allegedly framed him by planting a gun in his car.

In 2006, Fitzgibbons—an infectious disease specialist and former chief of staff at Western Medical Center—was arrested in the hospital parking lot after police found a pair of black gloves and a handgun in his car. Police questioned Fitzgibbons and searched his car after an anonymous 9-1-1 call claimed that the doctor had brandished the gun in traffic.

DNA evidence from the gloves and gun exonerated Fitzgibbons, and he was never charged.

However, the arrest followed a series of disagreements between Fitzgibbons and the leadership of Integrated Healthcare Holdings Incorporated (IHHI), which owned the Santa Ana hospital. Fitzgibbons and his attorney—Ted Mathews—alleged that IHHI's then-CEO, Bruce Mogel, had framed Fitzgibbons in an effort to silence him.

Specifically, Mathews said that the frame was part of Mogel's attempt to "humble" Fitzgibbons after the doctor won a legal victory over IHHI in June 2006.

During the trial, former IHHI President Larry Anderson testified that Mogel had instructed him to create a $10,000 contract for a "scary guy" named Mikey Delgado immediately after Fitzgibbon's legal victory. The contract was for unnecessary work on the health system's website. In his testimony, Anderson said he realized after Fitzgibbons was arrested that the contract was actually for the frame. Mathews told the jury that the $10,000 was used to "[get] Dr. Fitz set up."

IHHI's board learned of the $10,000 contract during Anderson's deposition in 2008. Instead of firing Mogel, the board awarded him an eight-month consultancy worth $43,750 per month, Mathews says. This showed that IHHI board "knew what Mogel did to Dr. Fitzgibbons," Mathews told the jury, adding, "They ratified it, and they gave him a golden handshake goodbye."

The jury ultimately decided that IHHI acted with "malice, oppression, or fraud against Dr. Fitzgibbons." It ordered the hospital to pay the doctor $5.2 million for emotional distress and $500,000 in punitive damages (Campbell, Orange Country Register, 2/13; Campbell, Orange Country Register, 2/8).

Concept # 3 Treating physicians as commodities rather than assets

According to Investopedia.com a commodity is: A basic good used in commerce that is interchangeable with other commodities of the same type. Commodities are most often used as inputs in the production of other goods or services.

This is how we believe most non-physician managers used to perceive physicians in the health care cycle. The best way to value physicians is by their RUVs.

There is no better way to illustrate the concept of "physicians as commodities" than the "hospitalist". The "hospitalist" is a concept that was introduced not long ago, and was a very new one for the medical community. The young hospitalist groups, usually small and formed by a few internists and family practice physicians, received some financial help from hospitals. The goal was to help the group to establish themselves and operate until they could become financially self-sufficient.

Here we are 15 years later, and hindsight makes it clear that the goal of financial independence was an unrealistic one at best. Hospitalists were working very long shifts and seeing high numbers of patients in an effort to decrease bed days stay and keep the re-admit rate low. It was not unusual for a hospitalist to follow 22-28 patients a day. This nightmare scenario was created because the income of a self-sufficient hospitalist group could not support enough hospitalists to do the tasks at hand.

Over the past 15 years things have changed for hospitalists, but not because managers are visionaries. Rather, changes have occurred merely because of the financial pressure felt by hospitals when they incur penalties for longer bed day stays, high infection rates, and other criteria well-known to you.

Innovators would have foreseen the benefit of a well-financed and well- staffed hospitalist program in busy hospitals. It was the physicians hospitalists for the most part, who promoted their cause with thick-minded hospital administrators to get to the current situation, where hospitalists work 12 hour shifts with a load of 12-15 patients.

Well, in the early days of becoming hospitalists the hours and work load were enough to burn out the average hospitalist in 2 to 3 years. And because hospitalists are commodities, they were being cycled every 2 to 3 years. This became a trend, especially when hospitals started realizing the benefit of hospitalist programs and wanted to be in charge of their own home grown programs.

The recognition on the part of managers that physician "churn" worked for the bottom line was communicated, in a way, to recruiters. Management would convey to the recruiters that their efforts should focus on picking up physicians who had recently completed their residency and had been accepted into fellowship programs. If the fellowship were to begin 2 years from their graduation from residency, the hospital could pick them up as independent contractors with no benefits. The hospital would have them for 2 years and just about the time that these young physicians burned out, it was time for them to move on to their fellowship. They were a commodity and they were replaced every 2 years - sooner if they burned out earlier.

That system did not work. Hospital management began to realize that a career hospitalist, with an exemplary track record well-known by specialists and ER doctors, and who has roots in the local community, is actually an asset. This type of hospitalist knows the system, facilitates communication in any number of ways, and on many occasions is able to avoid bottlenecks in the system by planning his or her day around them. This skill is developed over years of practice in the same hospital, and it has important value to the hospital and its patients. It cannot be measured by RUVs.

This type of skilled hospitalist is an asset. It takes time and hard work to develop beyond residency, and accumulate the training that leads to excellent medical skills.

The case with managers now is "better late than never" in their understanding of the importance of treating physicians as assets rather than commodities. In so doing, they have shifted their hiring practices. Now when they need to hire a medical director of a large hospitalist group, hospital administrators tend to select an experienced physician who is a long-time resident with roots in the local community; a physician who is already known to the community's physicians.

Those medical directors receive higher compensation than their RUVs, many times referred to as the "medical director stipend". Now hospital management recognizes that they have value that is worth more than their actual RUVs. Simply put, these medical directors have been upgraded from commodity status to an asset status.

What is so amazing is that in this day and age there are still hospitals and hospitalist groups (that answer mostly to stock holders), that treat the hospitalist physician as a commodity. What is even more amazing to us is that the health industry with its major players, Medicare being the largest, has not learned much from the history of the hospitalist. They continue to treat physicians as a commodity. They facilitate physician burnout by the constant tactical implementation of new regulations that lack strategic vision and aim at raiding savings, while eroding the rank of the most valuable "asset" in the health industry: the physician.

Concept # 4: The Insight Deprived Manager

I am going to suggest categorizing managers into two categories, those who have insight, and those who lack insight.

As we discussed earlier a manager is a "tactical policy implementer". They make sure that the policies that trickle down the rank of a health care entity are implemented. These policies frequently reflect the confused health care system that today is attempting to address the nation's health needs.

But, just like delivering a diagnosis of dementia or cancer to a patient and his or her family, it has to be done with insightful manner. Implementing trickle down policies has to be done with an excellent insight. A manager who lacks insight and understates the position of a local physician in the community is likely to come across as rigid, distant, and disconnected. This manager will be seen as a corporate suit, not an insightful leader.

This is the perfect time to ask yourself a simple question, "Am I working with corporate suits, or insightful leaders?" The absence of insightful leaders in your health care entity is likely to increase the risk of burnout among the physicians.

This is also the time to answer this question: "Am I treated like an asset or a commodity at my work?" We believe if you are treated as a commodity you are at a higher risk of burnout.

Concept #5 CEO turnover increased in the past few years

Because the cornerstone of executive/physician relationships can involve a lack of trust and understanding, it doesn't help that executive turnover makes developing relationships that much harder. CEO turnover in healthcare remains one of the highest rates recorded in the past 15 years. In 2014, the rate of hospital

CEO turnover decreased to 18 percent from the 20 percent recorded in 2013.

The American College of Healthcare Executives (ACHE) has tracked hospital CEO turnover since 1981. The 18 percent turnover rate matches what was seen in 1999 and 2009. In 2013, CEO turnover hit a high of 20 percent. In 2012, it was 17 percent, while it lingered at 16 percent in 2011 and 2010.

Again, an article in Becker's Hospital Review shed some light on the issue; "As our data show, elevated turnover among hospital CEOs seems to be a feature of the current healthcare environment," says Deborah J. Bowen, FACHE, CAE, ACHE's president and CEO. "The continuing trend of consolidation among organizations, the increasing demands on chief executives to lead in a complex and rapidly changing environment, and retirement of leaders from the baby boomer era may all be contributing to this continuing higher level of change in the senior leadership of hospitals."

There may be a silver lining to this high rate of turnover. B.E. Smith, the national healthcare executive search firm, is suggesting to its healthcare clients that they strongly consider changing the way they manage, including "development of leadership skills that reflect the changing demands and need for broad leadership integration," and the building of teams "that can operationalize strategic plans across aligned entities and induce significant change."

If hospital leadership were to heed the recommendation for leadership integration and the building of teams, physicians might finally find a meaningful place at the leadership table. If management were to consider physicians as important resources of information on patients, front-line revenue collection and patient perception of quality care, hospitals might end up actually being more responsive to patient needs, and more inclusive of physician's goals and objectives in health care.

Concept #6 The characteristics of the successful health care CEOs

The high turnover of healthcare CEOs over the past 15 years, and the crushing increase of reimbursement, government and regulatory changes have posed unique challenges for hospitals seeking to fill the chair in the C-suite. Physicians are the heart and soul of any hospital system and integrating them into leadership is not a maybe, it is now a must. Finding a forward-thinking, inclusive, collaborative executive who can also lead is a challenge of Herculean proportions. However, we do know the characteristics that effective leaders need to exhibit:

- Development of leadership skills that reflect the changing demands and need for broad leadership integration
- An understanding of the need for clinical integration

- Ability to successfully achieve physician alignment and participation, partnering with physicians on strategic goals
- The successful CEO will encourage, both through example and written hospital policy, accountability regarding financial efficiency, patient satisfaction, and quality of care.
- Communicates regularly with hospital employees, physicians and clinical staff. Advises them regularly on status of hospital finances, ensures that the internal audiences know of any major personnel changes, merges, acquisitions etc, before it appears in the news.
- Encourages excellence in quality of care by communicating regularly, the hospital rankings in surgical site infections, infection control, cardiac care, falls prevention, patient satisfaction, Press Ganey, HCAHPS and other key quality indicators.
- A depth of experience, business intelligence and purchaser relationships.
- A philosophy that includes the hospital as part of a community or region, and that population wellness is key to its success, and part of new reimbursement formulas.
- An understanding of the regulatory pressures facing physicians today, including ICD-10 and HER, that increase costs, require staff training, and physical and technology changes in the practice.
- Collaborative skills that will facilitate the building of cross-functional teams.

- An ability to work with differing opinions and practice perspectives in order to optimize operations.

- An inclusive approach to strategic planning that includes all key operational functions, and gives physicians a seat at the planning table.

- Entrepreneurial and creative, with the ability to find new sources of revenue as the healthcare industry continues to change and evolve rapidly.

Concept # 7 Physicians are the Best Managers of Hospitals

The search for leaders is a never-ending process. Simply put, physicians are the best leaders of hospitals.

Amanda Goodall, senior research fellow at the IZA Institute in Bonn, Germany conducted a study to determine if physician-led hospitals were better hospitals. Goodall's study, published in the journal Social Science & Medicine, is considered the first evidence toward proving the long held belief that having physicians in leadership positions is valuable for hospital performance.

Goodall's study took the top 100 U.S. hospitals in each of three specialties – cancer, digestive disorders and cardiac care and surgery – as ranked by US News and World Report for 2009. She then researched the backgrounds of their chief executives. Of the top 100 cancer hospitals, 51 had chief executives who were qualified doctors; of the top 100 units for digestive disorders, 34 had medical chief executives; of the top 100 cardiac centers there were 37 physician leaders. Further, her study established that doctor-led hospitals had quality scores some 25% higher than other units.

Available statistics show that there are some 6,500 hospitals in the U.S. and only 235 are led by doctors. Clearly there is much more work to be done in achieving physician leadership.

The very regulations that are creating intense pressure for physicians today, may also be the impetus that gets them into the C-suite. More hospitals are hiring doctors as CEOs as reimbursement increasingly rests on clinical quality rankings. Organization growth and direction has to be more closely aligned with the clinical side of the house, if hospitals want to survive.

The American College of Physician Executives, which helps groom doctors for management and leadership roles, published a white paper in April titled, "The Value of Physician Leadership,". As reported in Modern Healthcare, the paper explains some of the reasons for the rise of physician executives. The redesign of clinical-care models aligning payment with clinical excellence and improved outcomes puts physicians "at the center of this stage," according to the paper, which was co-written by ACPE President and CEO Dr. Peter Angood and Susan Birk. "Physician leadership is critical to shepherd healthcare into the future, creating a delivery system grounded in better health and better healthcare at lower cost."

Some of the most prominent hospitals in the country have physician CEOs including New York-Presbyterian University Hospital of Columbia and Cornell, the Cleveland Clinic, Mayo Clinic and Johns Hopkins Medicine, among others. Modern Healthcare reported that, "Physicians see top management positions as a powerful perch for leading the drive for improved quality of care, patient safety and clinical efficiency," according to Dr. Gary Gottlieb, president and CEO of Partners HealthCare in Boston. "Physicians are pursuing management roles to a greater degree than before," he said. "They get the bug because they realize how they can make things better."

Concept #8 A road map to developing an insightful manager / excellent health care CEO from within your organization

Healthcare CEOs are leaving in record numbers, so one would think that most hospitals would have succession planning in place. Unfortunately, this is not the case, and in fact, it is one area in which hospitals fail. B.E. Smith reports that 64% of hospital executives say they have no succession planning. Even more rarely does it include physician leaders. However, it should. Selective hiring and effective succession planning are essential for stability at the helm. Let's look at some of the things that need to be in place to develop the leaders of tomorrow.

A: How do you find potential leaders in the organization and develop them into executives?

They exhibit the following characteristics of a "young" leader:

- Calm demeanor and they calm others in their presence
- Quiet confidence when they speak.
- Extremely confident in their abilities, but not egotistical or condescending.
- They are not afraid to a risk that will improve themselves or their organization
- These young leaders take initiatives, bring problems to a discussion along with potential solutions, and set high expectations for themselves for job performance.
- Flexible, listen to opinions of others, collaborate and delegate
- Articulate

B: Is it better to bring in leaders from the outside?

There may be situations in which bringing new leadership in from the outside is best, usually in a turn-around situation, or after a crisis. Organizations may feel that they do not have a culture that develops potential executives with the cross-functional talents needed to lead the organization. In some cases, a hospital needs a leader experienced in mergers and acquisition to lead them through future events. In these cases, the search team would be wise to pay attention to the characteristics listed above in Concept #6, where we discuss the characteristics of a successful healthcare CEO.

C: Does a healthcare executive need an MBA to be effective?

Not necessarily. This is an "all depends" answer, depending upon the training of the executive. For example, a Chief Medical Officer isn't apt to have an MBA and yet a Chief Financial Officer would be expected to have one. The Chief Nursing Officer should have advanced nursing degrees and certifications, but an MBA is not going to enhance their job performance. A CEO may or may not have an MBA, but they usually do hold an advanced degree of one type or another. Today's CEOs may hold degrees in healthcare administration, or as we are discussing here, they may be experienced physicians with multiple degrees.

D: Is it possible to help executives understand how physicians think?

Yes, it is possible, but difficult unless you are a physician. There are times when office or practice managers meet with senior executives to facilitate operational issues between the practice and the hospital. Most usually agreements are not reached because even though the manager was sent to represent the practice, hospital executives are not in the habit of making decisions with middle managers. Any decision that involves operations or the bottom line will wait until the executives can meet with the physician directly. Regardless of whether or not the C-suite executives think physicians are commodities, they do put stock in their input and will wait to receive it.

E: Does it improve a corporate culture when the CEO or other top leaders abandon micro-management and instead develop a leadership team to which they can delegate tasks?

There are some who would say that to say yes to this answer is to look through rose-colored glasses. However, the answer is yes and it is beginning to take place in health care. As CEOs and other top leaders undertake strategic planning initiatives, expansions, and/or mergers with other healthcare organizations, collaboration and smart leadership is growing. Those leaders who are myopic, narrow-minded and narcissistic are being left behind. All the factors that we have discussed so far in this chapter regarding integration, quality implementation and stable physician practices depend upon leaders who can delegate initiatives and then let go. Developing task forces, planning teams, quality control leadership groups and the like not only brings new ideas to the table, it also creates buy-in and ownership from middle management, and increases accurate communication to lower level employees.

F: Is it futile to concentrate on technology investment as the main tool to remain competitive, which is the trend today?

It's not futile, but it has to be balanced with patient care. I agree that maintaining technology is key to an organization's survival. A physician practice without EHR is going to find it extremely difficult, if not impossible, to keep up with ICD-10 and reimbursement documentation. A hospital whose emergency room cannot telephonically communicate with stroke specialists is going to leave reimbursement money on the table.

However, patient care must remain the priority. Digital bedside patient registration has many benefits, but it must not replace face-to-face contact and empathy with the patient. Advanced EMRs can be life-savers, but only if the physician remembers to connect with his or her patient while using the tablet.

G: Should CEOs focus on investing in human assets?

In a word: yes. In addition to the challenges of succession planning, and the need for new and innovative CEO skill sets, there is another challenge that is upon us, and that is the aging workforce. The Catch 22 here is that just as the aging Baby Boomers need healthcare in record numbers, they are also retiring from the healthcare workforce in record numbers, leaving a dangerous vacuum of skilled workers in their wake.

The younger workforce has different values than the Baby Boomers. They work faster; want faster promotions, and more money. They aren't as patient and they don't live or work by the same standards and traditions as the Baby Boomers. This also means that they may not be attracted to leadership positions. They value free time and therefore may be more aware of the importance of work-life balance than the generation before them.

Investing in human assets is the key to any successful hospital. After all, it is the human assets that care for, treat and hopefully cure the human patients.

H: Is there, or can there be, a road map to building bridges with the physician community?

In some hospital cultures it seems that difficult hospital/physician relationships are as old as the hospital itself. Hospitals want to make money and so do physicians. Each may believe that the other stands in the way of that goal. On call hours are always a point of contention, as is the hospital bringing in competing specialty groups to expand service. Hospital executives want to establish clear cut business objectives, while physicians want to build their practices and patient panel. Hospitals often want physicians to comply with policies and procedures for the greater good, while physicians feel like a round peg being forced into a square hole.

If there were to be a roadmap, the signs on the main highway would read as follows:

- Ask physicians for input, listen to it, and value it.
- Involve physicians in leadership and real decision making, not just symbolic positions.
- Support new physician practices, offering guarantees or other revenue support before spinning them off.
- Help to bring in new physicians to growing practices and support the search.
- Treat physicians as valued assets to the hospital, rather than commodities that bring in business.

I: Can physicians help with succession planning?

Absolutely. There are millions of talented physicians practicing in the U.S. today, and yet current estimates show that they represent only 14% of current C-suite hires. Hospitals that understand the value of physician leaders are creating roles for them in operational, strategic and even cultural initiatives. If you research some of these new positions, you will find titles like Vice President of Clinical Transformation, or Vice President of Informatics. The increased focus on patient satisfaction is a key driver in seeking physician leadership, as is meeting and exceeding quality indicators. Instituting training programs for physician leaders so that they can drive a culture of accountability, transparency and excellence is a forward thinking initiative and one that will go a long way toward meeting the many conflicting priorities in healthcare today.

Tips for Making Solid Hiring Decisions

To avoid mistakes in the hiring process, consider these five tips to avoid common pitfalls and review proven hiring strategies from real companies and advisers.

1. Hire for the future. Jim Johnston, a C-suite adviser, warns not to let hiring decisions be influenced by the past, according to CFO Magazine. Delaying the replacement of an ineffective key executive, hiring an executive who fits the past but not the future needs of the business, or selecting from a small pool of candidates consisting of only familiar faces are all hazards.

"Recognize that each time your company fills a spot on the senior team, it's a moment for creating the future of your company," Mr. Johnston said.

While retirement, resignation or letting employees go create the need to hire someone new, each is an opportunity to incorporate a new leader than can propel the business forward. Making the wrong choice, however, can be a huge setback.

According to Mr. Johnston, there are several key symptoms of executives who do not fulfill important leadership requirements. These include avoidance, delay, failure to delegate and always being reactive instead of proactive.

2. Seek out entrepreneurs. A successful entrepreneur, by nature, is someone who can lead, take risks, take on multiple responsibilities and think critically. Entrepreneurs represent many of the traits a powerful executive should have. However, it is important to have a balanced approach when adding those with an entrepreneurial mindset and experience.

According to ReadWrite, Spencer Gerrol, founder and CEO of research and design firm SPARK Experience Design, said adding an entrepreneur to the executive team will work out best if his or her personality and work style complements those of the other executives already onboard.

For example, someone who is a risk-taker might need a more cautious person to keep them in check, while an analytical person may benefit from working with someone who is exceptionally creative, Mr. Gerrol explained.

3. Choose and inform search consultants wisely. According to an article in Businessweek by Joseph Daniel McCool, author of

Designing Who Leads, it's important to know when a retained executive search firm should be used instead of other forms of recruitment. These include if your organization wants to recruit an executive who is already working for a competitor, an executive who is not currently seeking a new opportunity or if the search needs to be kept confidential.

Don't let cost-per-hire determine executive search decisions. According to Mr. McCool, many organizations choose the lowest-bidding recruiter to handle executive searches, with cost avoidance as the motivation.

It is also important to research outside consultants to prevent conflicts of interest. According to an article in the Harvard Business Review, executive search consultants may sometimes offer an exceedingly favorable recommendation for candidates they found or an overly skeptical view of those with whom they were not involved in sourcing.

Additionally, make sure to specifically request leadership diversity in candidates from the search consultant to ensure they possess a range of leadership traits and experiences, Mr. McCool suggests.

4. Compare data on executive candidates from past colleagues. According to the Harvard Business Review, candid insight on candidates from those who have experience working with them is invaluable. Vetting the views of a candidate's prior colleagues executive boards — while still maintaining confidential— can

yield informative and sometimes surprising results, the article said.

5. Don't have institutional amnesia. Improving the organization's future performance partially depends on ensuring lessons learned from past errors aren't forgotten. According to Mr. McCool, it is important to record the performance of external advisors to inform future search process decisions.

"Hiring organizations can begin to reduce cost, accelerate the search process and track results if they know which search consultants [external advisers] are engaging, how they're engaging them and why," he said.

Resources:

Becker's Hospital Review http://www.beckershospitalreview.com/hospital-management-administration/5-things-to-keep-in-mind-when-hiring-an-executive.html

3 Things Hospital Executives Don't Get About Physician Integration

Written by Heather Punke (Twitter | Google+) | December 04, 2013

http://www.beckershospitalreview.com/hospital-physician-relationships/3-things-hospital-executives-don-t-get-about-physician-integration.html

http://www.beckershospitalreview.com/hospital-physician-relationships/top-10-physician-complaints-of-2013.html

http://www.beckershospitalreview.com/hospital-management-administration/hospital-ceo-turnover-down-from-2013-s-record-high.html

Hospital CEO turnover down from 2013's record high

Written by Molly Gamble (Twitter | Google+) March 05, 2015

Integration and aligning across entities; Healthcare executive compensation is adapting to new leadership competencies

Written by Ayla Ellison (Twitter | Google+) | January 12, 2015

http://www.beckershospitalreview.com/compensation-issues/healthcare-executive-compensation-is-adapting-to-new-leadership-competencies.html

Hospitals hire more doctors as CEOs as focus on quality grows

By Andis Robeznieks | May 10, 2014

Modern Healthcare 50 Most Influential Physician Executives

Holden Leadership Center, University of Oregon

http://leadership.uoregon.edu/resources/exercises_tips/skills/leadership_characteristics

Andria Corso, founder of C3-Corso Coaching & Consulting, http://www.careerealism.com/qualities-emerging-leader/

8 THE NEED TO GROW

Health Care organizations need to grow to remain viable. These include facilities that treat patients, as well as insurance companies, organizations involved in the management of health care systems, and companies that manage only part of the system like those who provide imaging and other allied services. We do not need to prove that reality with published papers and studies, just look at the growth status of Kaiser-Permanente, Dignity health (previously Catholic health), Mayo Clinic and the Cleveland Clinic. Spend a little time researching the growth of Blue Cross and Blue Shield. Finally, look over the public financial statements of these institutions and you will get a rude awakening when you see the infra-structure expenditures that some of them have included in their 10 year plan. Many of these are duplicate services delivered by other healthcare entities in the same geographic area.

The new trend of making the hospital a center of health care delivery will contribute to increased rates of burnout in the work force. This is especially true if planners and business development "experts" continue to develop expansion strategies that look good on paper, but that have had no input from the physician body. The expectation that any plan or strategy developed in isolation from physicians will then be successfully implemented by them is misplaced and ill-conceived. It ignores the daily reality of these physicians.

I quote the following points from an excellent article: "The Inevitability of Physician Burnout: Implications for Interventions"

By Anthony Montgomery,

University of Macedonia, Greece

Published in "Science Direct" online June 2014 "

1- Hospitals are unique organizational environments where the degree to which professional roles are strongly embedded represent a significant barrier to change (Mintzberg, 1997).
2- Hospitals are organizations under considerable stress. For example, in the UK, surveys show that continuity of care for the patient is being compromised (Hawkes, 2012). This is not surprising when one considers that healthcare professionals are expected to handle structural changes and technical developments, required to be accessible, provide holistic patient-centered and patient-managed care, develop

their own evidence-based competence and achieve an appropriate balance between their work and private lives.

3- Without too much effort, the purpose of a hospital can become self-preservation and not healing, which is reinforced by the way that health care organizations can be organized in silos (Glouberman & Mintzberg, 2001).

4- The Institute of Medicine (IOM) in the US has repeatedly highlighted the link between patient safety and organizational culture (Institute of Medicine, 2001 and Kohn et al., 1999), and burnout has been identified as the crucial link between organizational culture and quality of care (Montgomery et al., 2013 and Montgomery et al., 2011a).

Hospitals are organizations that reinforce a pathogenic approach to health. Not surprisingly, this has dominated the way we think about, and implement, health care. "

If they cannot grow they will die

Healthcare entities need to grow. If they cannot they will die. If they die, what will happen to patients?

It is important to recognize that these entities grow at the expense of smaller physician practices. As systems merge with and acquire other systems, physician practices experience tremendous displacement. Indeed, small practices may someday disappear altogether, either through acquisition by a larger system, going bankrupt because of these market changes, or becoming employees of the hospital or healthcare system instead of running their own practice, despite the fact that both parties may not be ready for that union.

This unfit "seed" of a business model that is being sown across the US is one of the main issues that can feed into physicians' burnout. Furthermore, it is easy to see from the following case study, that the success of this model is very questionable in many markets.

This case study was published by the "Commonwealth Fund" in June of 2009. It is an in-depth look at the Kaiser-Permanente experience which, for many in the business, serves as the most viable healthcare business model available today. Certainly the policy makers charged with "saving Medicare" and many other major players trying to address the healthcare crisis in the US are trying to copy this model. The case study is as follows:

Kaiser Permanente: Bridging the Quality Divide with Integrated Practice, Group Accountability, and Health Information Technology

Douglas McCarthy, Kimberly Mueller, and Jennifer Wrenn Issues Research, Inc.

Kaiser Permanente—comprising the Kaiser Foundation Health Plan, Kaiser Foundation Hospitals, and Permanente Medical Groups in eight regions—is the largest nonprofit integrated health care delivery system in the United States.

The successful evolution of this organizational structure in a competitive marketplace has required a close partnership between managers and physicians supported by a culture of physician group accountability for quality and efficiency.

An overarching agenda for achieving excellence focuses on high-impact health conditions, provides goal-oriented tools to analyze population data, proactively identifies patients in need of intervention, supports systematic process improvements, and promotes collaboration between patients and professionals to improve health.

Central to this effort is KP Health Connect, a comprehensive health information system that integrates an electronic health record with the tools to support physicians in delivering evidence-based medicine, coupled with a robust online patient portal that enhances members' access to and involvement in their care.

The Kaiser Permanente model of integrated group practice has the advantage of having evolved over seven decades, but it may not be easy to replicate today. During the 1980s and 1990s, Kaiser sought to expand in several new regions, but only two (Georgia and the Mid-Atlantic) proved successful. Researchers who studied the North Carolina experience found that a combination of political, economic, and organizational factors contributed to the plan's withdrawal from that state. They concluded that realizing the potential of this model in new markets requires a "conjuncture of several supportive conditions," such as gaining a critical mass of members to support the delivery of a full scope of services that can be internalized within the multispecialty group. Doing so may depend in large part on whether purchasers offer and reward consumers for selecting better-value options. (End case study)

Adapting the Kaiser-Permanente Model is like training an army

As I look into the future through my "Magic Ball" I can imagine easily the potential benefits of adapting a model like Kaiser-Permanente. However, what I also see happening when pursuing this course, is a definite erosion of the physician work force from burnout.

My magic ball also shows me that the attempt to adapt this model harkens back to other failed initiatives in the geo-political world, namely, creating trained armies in third world countries after bringing down an unwanted regimen. These failed attempts are usually undertaken with the assumption and expectation that the newly created army will be able to move in and take over for the US trained armed forces when they pull out. I cannot recall a single success. To make matter worse, the process always involves spending enormous funds to create militia of inexperienced native mercenaries that further devastate the very country they were meant to save and protect.

Building an army is about building a culture. Having state of the art equipment, excellent advisors, and very well trained generals are a start, but they cannot become the United States Army. They do not have the years of experience, nor the long standing military culture that creates the strength of the US armed forces.

How does that relate to the Kaiser-Permanente experience?

The answer is very simple. It took Kaiser-Permanente 70 years to develop its culture. It is not possible to replicate this in other health care entities in a mere 5 or 10 years. In other words, Kaiser-Permanente is not a burger joint that can be franchised.

The Wrong Philosophy

This paragraph is going to be, to say the very least, "provocative". I am myself not sure of the ultimate answer to this dilemma, but I feel it should be brought out in the open for more discussion.

The provocative question I pose is this, "What could possibly be the most prevalent "wrong philosophy" in healthcare today, which should not be, but is, accepted as a matter of fact?"

The provocative answer is: The most prevalent "wrong philosophy" in healthcare today is the mixing and mingling of physicians' roles as diagnostician, disease and sickness healers with the function of public health officials.

I am aware of many studies that speak for the influence of

physicians on the behavior of their patients. I am also well aware of the inherit benefits and advantages that come with using physician-patient interactions to promote public health issues. I also realize that the most important factor behind this idea is that public health officials gain "free and cheap" access to the patient through their doctor.

I will admit that this model did work well in pediatrics to improve certain issues such as immunization. However, it has not been as effective in requiring students to have their vaccines up to date before starting pre-school.

The problem with the physician-as-public-health-conveyer philosophy is the desire on the part of administrators to roll it out on the national level, making health care entities responsible for the "health of the nation". These policy makers are making the presumption that this equation will save healthcare dollars if only it can be implemented nationwide. The equation looks like this: large hospital and healthcare systems + convincing their physicians to advocate for public health issues + physician-to-patient influence = millions and millions of healthcare dollars saved.

Taking advantage of the physician-patient relationship is one of the core arguments of the success stories within the Kaiser-Permanente model. This is one of the reasons it is advocated for as a model for the new national health care system wherein large health care organizations are in charge of the "health of the nation". The argument is that these entities are very good at diagnosis and treatment, so they should be just as good at changing people's minds and convincing them to choose and follow healthier life-styles.

Now ask yourself these questions and use them as a road map to your own answers. We did not research the literature for answers, but you may want to do so:

1- Is mixing the role of a physician diagnosing and treating illness with the role of a public health official a good use of the physician's time?

2- Is mixing the role of a physician with the role of a public expert a good use of the physician time?

3- Do smokers quit smoking because they are influenced by their physician's advocacy or by other factors?

4- Do people elect to lose weight, begin exercising or develop an active lifestyle due to the recommendations of their physicians during their annual visit?

5- Are public figures, celebrities, and public advertising campaigns less effective than the physician-patient interaction in promoting behavioral changes?

6- Most of your patients have researched their own signs and symptoms and have a list of a differential diagnoses of their conditions before they come to see you. Indeed, some of them already have a "request list" of laboratory and radiology studies that should be conducted - according to their research - and they demand to have them. The internet has changed everything in the practice of medicine. Do you think that the information you would give most of your patients in a printed handout is going to be more believable to them than that they can for themselves on the internet?

I quote here a paragraph from Stanford Medicine published online. I leave it up to you to draw your own conclusions, and decide for yourself if you want to assume the role of "The Utopian Physician":

How Physicians address obesity may affect patients' success in losing weight

Emily Hite on February 18th, 2014

"For some patients, the need to begin a weight-loss program to lower health risks connected with obesity is urgent. But losing weight and keeping it off for the long term can be a challenging journey for a person – and patient-doctor conversations about weight loss can be complex.

A study recently published online in Preventive Medicine looked at the way patients perceive their physicians' attitudes about obesity, and the patients' change in weight following the delivery of weight-loss advice. For their work, the researchers conducted Internet-based surveys in 500 adults with a body-mass index of 25 or more.

As explained in a Johns Hopkins release:

The participants were asked, "In the last 12 months, did you ever feel that this doctor judged you because of your weight?" Twenty one percent of participants said they believed they had been.

Further, 96 percent of those who felt judged did report attempting to lose weight in the previous year, compared to 84 percent who did not. But only 14 percent of those who felt judged and who also discussed weight loss with their doctor lost 10 percent or more of their body weight, while 20 percent who did not feel judged and also discussed shedding pounds lost a similar amount.

"Negative encounters can prompt a weight loss attempt, but our study shows they do not translate into success," study leader Kimberly Gudzune, MD, MPH, an assistant professor in the Division of General Internal Medicine at the Johns Hopkins University School of Medicine, said in the release. "If we are their advocates in this process — and not their critics — we can really help patients to be healthier through weight loss."

TOO BIG TO FAIL

What happens once health care is delivered through very large health care organizations that span many states?

The size, shape and efficacy of the health care market is what determines patient outcomes when the system is strained. I present this doomsday scenario in a "cheesy" Hollywood Fiction Short Story:

The scene is San Francisco in the year 2040. There are only two very large health care organizations in existence. One delivers care to the population of the Bay area and San Jose and carries the "imaginative" name of "University of California Health Care Systems". The second organization delivers care from the East Bay area to Sacramento and is named "Kaiser-Federal Health Care Alliance".

In this story, the CEO of the "University of California Health Care System" dies unexpectedly during a routine robotic colonoscopy. The cause is discovered to be the failure of a computer chip manufactured in India rather than China, which is known to have reliable electronic manufacturing.

A new CEO is chosen from a large pool of very talented scientists who are considered rising stars. He is futuristic in his visions for the large health organization. His intriguing concepts and incredible charisma fires up the board of directors and they carry out a restructuring of the entire health system.

This approach has always worked for the "University of California Health Care System". They have always allowed a select group of their brightest minds, those who chose leadership over academic achievements, to become leaders armed with extensive administrative hands-on experience. They also gave leadership positions to a few "stars" holding administrative and leadership degrees from the best business schools in the country. Under the leadership of such CEOs, the system was able to move leaps and bounds ahead of the most promising organization to dominate the health care market in the Bay Area in the early years of the 21st century. At the same time, what was known as "Kaiser-Permanente", was forced to move to the East Bay area, and after infrastructure changes and mergers they changed their name to "Kaiser-Federal Health Care Alliance".

The excellent "Kaiser-Permanente" leadership development program worked well for them through the 20th century. It consistently produced solid leaders who successfully implemented the economic/public health approach toward health care. Their model became the one that the federal government adapted in the early 21st century to solve "The Medicare Problem".

The Kaiser Permanente program of leadership preparation relied on identifying all the physicians with leadership potential and channeling them through a unique, proven, and quite superb system of leadership development. These potential leaders were trained, while at the same time were gradually eliminated from advancing in the hierarchy of leadership ladder. Those who were eliminated had already developed exceptional management skills and had assumed different management tasks in the organization. These potentials leaders who remained in the development pool were considered to be the "cream of the crop" and at the top were 3 or 4 highly trained, loyal, and exceptional CEOs-to-be from which to choose when needed.

That same incredible system that was perfect for the mature organization that they were, did not serve Kaiser-Permanente well in a rapidly changing health care market. The new health care world relied on the ability to develop innovative technology as much as it relied on consuming it.

Fast-forward to the year 2047. The innovative changes implemented by the "University of California Health Care System" were at least 15 years ahead of their time, and did not serve the year 2047 very well. The system lost money. Even though it was not a very large sum when compared to the total operating budget, it was enough to produce a ripple effect because of the very small margins both they and Kaiser operated on. Cuts in services and staff were necessary. Millions of people could not be cared for by the system and their employers chose to shift to the only other system in the area," Kaiser-Federal Health Care Alliance". Even though it could take hours to travel to the East Bay area, these people felt they had no choice. They needed to receive healthcare.

Public confidence in the "University of California Health Care System" began to erode. In a domino effect, this led to precautionary shifts on the part of large Far East manufacturing companies who held international health insurance contracts with the University system. These companies decided to shift their specialized care to the satellite "Mayo Clinic Health System" located in the Arabic Gulf Peninsula.

As a bit of background, the manufacturers found it very expensive to keep high-tech, specialized medical available in their own countries. They knew it was much more economical to contract with the "University of California Health Care System" for complex therapies and procedures for their employees in San Francisco, Los Angeles, Orange County, and San Diego. Those workers would be brought to the University system aboard "Cruise Ships of The Republic of China". The ships had been converted into enormous floating medical convalescent centers where employees recovered from their very specialized procedures at the centers of excellence of "University of California Health Care System".

Decades ago the heavily funded, poorly envisioned "Cruise Ships of The Republic of China" failed. However, their venture assets were not a complete loss. They had put their ships to innovate use, and it grew to be the largest fleet in the world to offer such a medical service, specifically tailored to servicing the health needs of Far East Asia.

Going back to the ripple effect in progress in the University system, losing the Far East Asian contracts shakes the system, and California employers start to leave the "University of California

Health Care System". However, the other smaller systems in California cannot handle the sudden flood of patients.

Contrary to the early years of the 21st century, services have been consolidated very efficiently, waste has been almost eliminated, and this has naturally eliminated any unnecessary extra capacity.

 Now the system is in jeopardy and the federal government has to inject money to allow the gigantic system to keep running, take care of citizens, and prevent major layoffs. The government bails out the failing health care system. (End Scene)

This is, of course, only a Hollywood fantasy. It is a fictional, and very unrealistic version of an exaggerated future in health care, for the sole purpose of entertaining you. However, our point is not fictional, it is very real. The point is "they may get too big to fail".

Not for Profit does not Equal "Green" nor "Consumer Friendly"

Most of us agree that if stock holders invest in a company they want profit; they are not investing simply to advance a noble cause. If this were the case, you would never see investments in tobacco companies. However, the contrary is true because tobacco companies are very profitable. It is extremely difficult to find a fund or investment firm that does not invest in a tobacco company.

What happens if profits shrink and dividends decline? Stock holders and investors move their money to another investment.

That says it all for for-profit health care entities. They have to continue to be profitable and increase their return on investment to continue to be attractive for future investment. A warning comes with that premise; there is only so much you can do to achieve efficient operations. When you have cut everything you can but find you need to cut more, sometimes the only thing left to cut is medical care for the patients.

But what about not for-profit health care entities?

1- They have to keep growing to be able to compete with the enlarging for-profit organizations.
2- They do not have to pay federal taxes so they are shielded to some extent from management inefficacies and wasteful administrative spending.

Regardless of those factors, if they don't watch their operations and keep an eagle eye on their finances, sooner or later they will reach the same point as for-profit organizations. They will have to cut medical services to patients and payments to physicians in order to stay competitive and preserve money for growth and survival.

For the most part the biggest competitors for health care non-profits aren't other for-profit or non-profit organizations. In our opinion, the biggest threat to survival for non-profit health care organizations is that they are destined to succumb to the laws of "Self-Preservation". Let us explain what we mean by that.

By their nature, many non-profits have a culture of "do good". Management and employees subscribe to the concept of, "We can do this because we are non for-profit and it is for the common good".

Most of them believe this and subscribe to the philosophy wholeheartedly.

That means a whole culture of industry that most of the management and employees may subscribe to the concept: "We can do this because we are non for-profit and it is for the common good".

However, once one of these organizations moves to" Self-Preservation" mode they will loose track of the vision that they were established with. The "do good" mantra becomes " what we do is for the common good" and the leadership scrambles to save the organization and cut wherever possible to improve the financial situation. Employee and physician morale begins to decay as leadership refuses to buy new medical equipment, pay more for on-call, and eschew annual raises. Employee thank you lunches, recognition dinners and food at meetings are all cancelled. Travel for training is nixed and everyone's favorite free Thanksgiving turkeys are no longer handed out. Employees and physicians eventually begin to ask, "If leadership is no longer interested in doing "good", what kind of organization are we working for?"

This is merely my observation and anecdotes based on people who have lived through such an experience in their hospital. I do not have any formal research to support whether our overall impression is true or false. I leave it up to you to make your own observations and you're your own conclusions as you look around your own health care organization.

I included this piece to serve as a brain tease!

9 THE PHYSICIAN'S SPOUSE

As a physician spouse you are part of a living organism called a physician career. This organism continues to live as long as the physician continues to practice medicine. The following concepts are different lenses through which you can observe this living organism, and see it from different angles.

Concept #1 The Healer

Your spouse is a healer; not just a professional.

Your spouse is driven, smart, dedicated, ambitious, but so too are many other professionals in other careers and high paying jobs, like technology, finance, accounting and management.

Going to medical school was not "Plan B" if your spouse could not make it as a stock broker, or become a very successful real estate agent. No, going to medical school was Plan A, and there was no back up "plan B". The plan went like this: Work hard for years preparing as pre-med, pass the MCAT, and apply to med school. If the initial application process was not successful, then go back to fattening the resume by completing other master degrees, PHD, publishing research, or working for years in a research lab.

Actually, you may know several successful professionals, with very high incomes, who elected not to go to medical school. They decided wisely that the financial reward of medicine was not worth the time they would have to spend getting there. Some of them may refer to themselves as "economically smarter than going to med school".

Your spouse was not blind to the sacrifice, or the financial consequences of pursuing a medical career.

He or she chose to be a healer, and you may have been attracted to him or her because of that. Well also because, needless to say, your spouse is beautiful or handsome, smart, well-spoken, and likes your cat or dog.

If you did not have a very good understanding of the "healer" part, this is the perfect time to brush up on it.

According to many studies spousal support is a major factor in combating burnout syndrome. Those physicians who enjoy spousal support are less likely to develop burnout and less likely to be unhappy with their careers.

The easiest way to think of "healing powers" is to think of video game characters. These characters need their healing powers re-charged on a regular basis. They get drained while helping others.

To recharge to full power, they need time and a fairy with the ability to radiate positive energy. During recharge, the video game character is less interactive, slower, less attentive and engaging. In your life, you are that fairy, and the time allowed for recharge is frequently dictated by you.

Now you know the simple rules for recharging the healing powers, and it is all in your hands.

You may say, and if you do it's perfectly natural, "I too am beaten and weary by the end of the day. My positive energy has been zapped. I need recharging myself." All other spouses are in the same boat. This can be true whether you have married a financial advisor, programmer, or a plumber. You married a healer, and because of that you have responsibility to keep him or her recharged, keep the family going, and you also bear some responsibility toward your spouse's patients. This is the package you signed up for when you became a physician's spouse.

This is why a physician's life style is a living organism.

Concept # 2 the Shielder

The "Healer" is also a "Shielder"

Your spouse will shield you from the day's sad stories. Occasionally he or she may tell you a success story. If your spouse doesn't tell you about the work day, do not assume it is because everything is great. For a physician, misery, suffering and sad stories are a daily occurrence. These stories come home with your physician spouse every day. They may cause your spouse to be silent and introspective, less attentive and disengaged from the family. Occasionally the sadness and suffering may surface as a casual minimalistic statement like, "I had a harder day than usual today. I am going to watch TV for a while and then join you for dinner."

It is definitely upsetting when your spouse ignores the effort you made to prepare a home cooked meal, or score tickets to a long awaited concert. You can lovingly convince your spouse to eat with the family or go to the concert, saying "Socializing will make you feel better." You may not realize the full benefits that your spouse experiences from your support, but you may feel his or her negative energy dissipating throughout the evening.

Your physician spouse's intuitive shielding behavior comes either from being an inexperienced physician, or from being a physician who is inexperienced in the art of recharging his or her batteries. Not talking about the day's misery, success or frustrations, internalizing and pushing through it have been built into your physician's psyche through the many stages of his or her training and career.

The Burnout rate is high in medical school, residency, and later on during practice. That is because traditionally the training has been: suck it up, keep going, there are many people to help and they are counting on you. Shove your feelings deep inside, and keep going. Physicians were always taught that expressing natural insecurities means weakness, and asking for support means you are "not tough enough for the job".

As a spouse of a physician, you are part of the team taking care of the patients. You are in charge of recharging your spouse's "healing powers". You are also in charge of getting your spouse to re-learn how to talk about their work day. You have to discover how to take down the shield that has been so carefully erected by your "shielder" physician spouse.

Concept # 3 The Physician Spouse's Internal Positive Energy

As a person you have limited capacity for internal positive energy. Therefore you must use it wisely as you recharge your physician spouse's "healing energy".

If you cannot listen to many sad stories of the day, do not spend your internal positive energy forcing yourself to extract these stories from your spouse. Humans are wired differently, and not all of us can handle the same level of human suffering. Of course it will help your spouse when he or she talks about the day, but this should not come at the cost of a large amount of your internal positive energy.

Focus the expenditure of your positive energy on maintaining a balance between what you need to keep going happily in your day, and giving your spouse what s/he needs to recharge.

With that said, your first task should be to know yourself when it comes to your spouse's medical practice. What can you handle to hear, and what can't you handle? Once you have mastered your own internal limits and the energy necessary for them, direct the rest of your internal positive energy into the things that best recharge your spouse.

Concept #4 The Devaluation of the Healer

One of the most devastating variables to a physician's career is the gradual loss of "Healing powers". Unfortunately, this is a double edge sword that cuts both ways. It is a consequence of burnout syndrome, as the afflicted physician feels less and less fulfilled by practicing medicine. It is at the same time a cause of burnout syndrome, imposed on physicians by the changing health care system, increased administrative work, and a re-imbursement system that rewards the technician rather than the healer.
By reminding your spouse of the "healing powers" the profession encompasses, you are helping to restore one of the pillars that defined his or her medical career. By doing so, you are also

keeping balance in your marriage. You can deliver this important reminder directly to your spouse by acknowledging (maybe once a month, when you are close emotionally), that he or she is a remarkable person, and you greatly appreciate the fact he or she is contributing to healing people. This recognition is as powerful a recharger as listening to your spouse's stories of suffering. So, if medical stories are not your cup of tea, you do have other options that will recharge your spouse and maintain a healthy marriage, while at the same time expending much less positive energy on your part.

You can also reinforce the important healing that your physician spouse practices in indirect ways. For example, as appropriate, you can tell the kids that their Mom or Dad is a healer. Inevitably they will begin to ask their parent what it means to be a healer and why it is important. Your spouse will know those good, kind messages came from you.

Use your imagination, and be clever. But beware, do not overuse the healing power recharging statement too much; it will lose its healing powers!

Concept # 5 It is an epidemic

I hope that as the spouse of a physician, you will read this book in its entirety. Burnout among physicians is not only growing, it is a problem of epidemic proportions. No one is immune to it. Reading this book will prepare you to identify the symptoms of burnout and begin to address them.

If your spouse is a physician that takes Medicare or accepts private insurance, these factors by themselves will automatically expose him or her to many variables responsible for developing some degree of burnout syndrome.

If you can only read parts of this book, here are some important things you need to know. If your spouse is exhibiting any combination of the signs and symptoms below, you should seriously consider discussing with your spouse, the fact that he or she may be suffering from burnout syndrome.

1- When your spouse responds to questions, it is frequently a diminished yes or no.

2- Your spouse likes to spend more time alone to re-charge.

3- Your spouse's sleeping habits are changing; spending more time watching TV before able to fall asleep, waking up frequently at night, snoring due to new weight gain.

4- Your spouse frequently feels fatigued, including the weekends.

5- Your spouse is avoiding socialization with friends and neighbors.

6- Your spouse is becoming cynical.

7- Your spouse has lost his or her sense of humor.

8- Your spouse is not interested in intimacy.

9- Your spouse feels distant.

10-You spouse's eating habits have changed significantly.

Before you start blaming yourself or thinking you have done something wrong to cause this behavior, start learning more about burnout syndrome. Then concentrate on the positive things you can do to help.

Concept # 6 the Lover

You have the powers of a lover; those powers can heal many of the psychological cuts and scratches your spouse encounters during the course of a day. The power of a huge, snuggle and gentle loving words are immense.

Being a lover for the long term requires two people in the relationship. For it to thrive, the other person has to return your emotions. Otherwise, the outpouring of your heart will gradually become a feeling of resentment and rejections, and the fountain of love will dry up very quickly. Your biggest challenge when dealing with possible burnout syndrome as the spouse of a physician is the difficulty your physician spouse may have in openly communicating his or her emotions. The tendency to become inward focused, over-occupied with work, and distant may come across as a lack of interest in you and avoidance of emotional involvement. In reality, they are the perfect storm of symptoms for burnout syndrome.

Once again you may find the burden rests on you to embrace your spouse with bursts of love and hugs. It will be your responsibility to lavish him or her with patience and kindness in order to help your spouse heal the wounds that come from the daily practice of medicine. Never fear- ultimately you are going to win. Studies have shown that physicians with supportive spouses who manage to spend quality time together are the ones who are more immune to burnout syndrome. Indeed, this alone is one of the most important factors in the life of the well balanced physicians.

Your last task related to the concept of the Lover is to define what constitutes healing quality time as a couple. This is a little different from what you have defined as quality "couple time" so far. It may be harder, unilateral, and like a prescription medication, may take a long time to work. This prescription has to be compounded just for the two of you. Only the two of you can figure out the most important elements in your "quality couple time" prescription. This is not an over the counter medication.

Concept # 7 the Hope

If you are feeling that you are losing hope, then burnout syndrome is already in an advanced stage. Our book is not enough, and both you and your spouse need to seek professional help from a psychologist. Frequently it is harder to get your physician spouse to proceed with therapy, especially when it is a male physician. Your spouse may have already progressed deep into the depersonalization stage, where most of his or her identity is defined with how hard he or she works. Your spouse feels that he or she is an exemplary physician, and there is nothing wrong. The natural conclusion for your spouse is that there is no need for intervention.

In these moments you may feel that there is no hope of a positive outcome. Hope starts to leave you; it feels as though it is fading away, turning its back on your relationship and your marriage. You run out of positive energy, and then you run out of energy all together. You may feel empty on the inside with ongoing, unexplained mental anguish. Hope is gone.

You are 100% wrong; there is still so much hope. It is even more important to know that the spouse you married is still in there somewhere, not dead, just dormant. Your spouse has given up on the "Healer", the "Shielder", the "Lover", and the "Hope embracer". He is a mechanical doctor.

Remember, hope is not gone for you.

Hope is salvaging the "Healer" that you married.

You have to be the "Hope embracer" and carry on the torch

salvaging all the investments the two of you have made together; financial, personal, and emotional.

You can salvage most of it and bring hope back, but things cannot stay the same.

Concept # 8 the Diagnostician

You do not need to be a professional to diagnose burnout syndrome. Being a spouse with natural intuition is more than enough to detect the problem. This could be the most important step moving forward, because once your intuition leads you to suspect burnout, it will be easy to recognize the signs and symptoms. It will be a relief to know that everything you see and sense from your spouse is not your fault; it is not something you have been doing. Once you are sure of your diagnosis, ask your spouse's friends and colleagues if they have observed changes in his/ her behavior, and if so, to describe the behaviors.

Ancillary personnel could also be sensing that "something has changed about the doctor"; he or she is a little less compassionate, a little less efficient, a little more irritable, a little less nice. They may have already decided to blame "tension in the marriage" for these subtle changes.

It is difficult to ask personnel these questions directly without irritating your spouse. One of the more practical ways to find out what is going on is to take advantage of an invitation to an office party, a lecture dinner, or similar event. Some of these are very boring to the non-medical guest. You will have to endure the pain of sitting through a scientific lecture for an hour or so. However, your patience (and resisting the urge to fall asleep) will be well worth the reward when you are able to ask all the questions you want about your spouse in an unassuming, non-threatening atmosphere. No one will be the wiser. They will perceive your questions as an attempt to be kind and sociable.

You may want to implement such a diagnostic approach years before you need to implement emergency interventions. Be an early diagnostician.

Concept # 9 the Child

Children are very intuitive and instinctive. They see things in a much simpler way than adults. They have a clear, simple view of life; it's black and white, good and bad, fun and boring. This is why if you are in doubt as to whether burnout syndrome is present in your spouse, and/or your marriage, ask your 8 year- old child this simple question: Do you want to be a doctor when you grow up? If the answer is no, then you should investigate further to determine whether or not your marriage is strained by the early stages of burnout syndrome.

You will know for sure that burnout syndrome is present in your marriage if one of your child's comments is:

1- Daddy spends most of the weekend writing notes.
2- Mommy does not want to play with me when she is back from work.
3- All that daddy does is watch TV.
4- Mommy is falling asleep when she is reading a story to me.
5- I can hear daddy talking on the cell phone at night. Sometimes he is loud and wakes me up.
6- Mommy's patients call her on her cell phone. She never lets me answer her phone.

How Are Spouses of Physicians Doing

A study published by Mayo Clinic in 2012 addressed the issue of being married to a doctor. The title of the study was, "The medical marriage: a national survey of the spouses/partners of US physicians."

It was a national survey and not limited to Mayo physicians. It included 1644 spouses or partners of physicians who were surveyed in 2011. Of those, 891 responded, which represents 54.2%, slightly more than half.

86.8% reported that they were satisfied with their relationship with their physician partners. Their satisfaction related directly to the time spent with their physician partners each day. There was a dose-response effect.

Despite their overall satisfaction, spouses and partners reported that their physician partners frequently came home irritable, too tired to engage in home activities, or preoccupied with work.

No professional characteristic of the physician's practice, like hours per week, specialty, or practice setting, impacted spouse/partner satisfaction. The only identified factor which correlated inversely with satisfaction was the number of nights on call per week.

Another paper published in 2004 tried to answer the same question of how physicians' wives are doing being married to a physician. Responses of 603 members of the American Medical Association Alliance indicated a high level of marital adjustment and overall satisfaction with work/life balance.

This adjustment was affected by:

1- Age of oldest child

2- Husband's work hours

3- Wife's work outside home.

It was proposed that, rather than the issue of the number of hours worked, the way in which couples treat each other when not at work most powerfully determined the quality of a contemporary medical marriage.

But there is more to the story:

What about divorce?

Let us compare divorce rates of physicians in the 1970s with those in the 1990s.

Divorce among Physicians in the 1970s and 1980s

This issue was examined in a paper published in JAMA in 1989. The data was aggregated from 1970s and 1980s US census data. The conclusion of the study was that things were good for physicians and their spouses, and that both male and female physicians have a lower tendency to divorce than other occupational groups, including other groups of professionals.

So what happened to Divorce among Physicians after the 1990s?

Divorce among Physicians after the 1990s

Multiple papers have been published documenting an increased rate of divorce among physicians. Here we refer to one paper that has been mentioned more frequently than other publications:

The Medical Marriage: A couple's Survival Guide. By Sotle in 1996. According to the publication, divorce rates are 10-20%

higher among physicians comparable to other groups.

In summary, physicians' divorce rate went from below average to above average after the early 1990s. Now you have to stop and think about this. You have to wonder what happened in one decade and try to make sense of it.

-The divorce rate of physicians has increased alarmingly since the 1990s.

-Yet physicians' spouses are more than 80% satisfied with their marriages.

-50% of the doctors may be suffering of an element of burnout syndrome.

What is the deal here?

After researching the subject, my best estimate is that burnout is responsible for the steep increase in the divorce rate. Not recognizing burnout early, lack of action on the part of managers when it is recognized early, lack of interest on the part of the medical community in addressing the issue; all have led to a build-up of internal strain on physicians' marriages.

What is so alarming to us is the sub- zero approach to not blaming the early stages of burnout syndrome for the damages we think they are causing.

I have to remind our readers that this is solely a conclusion on my part, based on the papers and data we have reviewed. But if I was even partially right, then this is a crisis that will eventually impact everyone in the next 10 years, as the loss of autonomy of physicians becomes the norm in medical practice. (When we say everyone we mean the general population that is 'patients".) I discuss the impact of burnout on the quality of medical care in more detail in other chapters.

At the end of this chapter I discuss a much more fun subject-having fun! I have provided a list of tools so that you can regularly, and pro-actively, freeze burnout syndrome in its early stages. Work, government legislation, insurance regulation and corporate policies are all variables that are out of your control. However, the tools that you have within your control have Nuclear Grade capabilities and you can count on them. They are tools that can help channel the power of your restorative love and internal positive energy into your spouse on a regular basis. The more you do, the more ingrained, and unconscious, positive behavior they become for your physician spouse.

Tools For Her:

It's the simple gestures that make the biggest impact- call them tiny acts of random kindness. It is being thoughtful, kind, and loving that keeps a relationship alive. Some men like to talk; others will never sit down and tell you how they feel. Keeping the lines of communication open may feel one-sided, but you have to keep trying so they won't shut down forever. You need open lines of communication so that your partner knows very clearly how much you love him.

For example: when you are watching Gray's Anatomy together, snuggle up to him, and whisper: Babe, I love that you are a doctor, and that you can heal people.

He will hear: I love you, I love the fact you heal people, I know you are the real deal. Gray's Anatomy is only a dramatization of doctors, but we both still like to watch it.

Other gestures include:

- Turn down his side of the bed and spray the pillows lightly with lavender.
- Make sure that the clothes he will want in the morning are on top when he opens the drawer, or in front when he opens the closet.
- If you leave for work first, or sleep in as he gets ready, prepare the coffee so it begins to brew when he gets up. (If your coffee maker has a timer!)
- Leave a small note in the kitchen, in his car, or in his briefcase, telling him that he is wonderful.
- Buy a special breakfast food that he can eat in the car and leave it for him on a nice plate.

- If you can, put his towels in the dryer to warm up while he is taking a shower.
- Send him a text saying "I love you" in the middle of the day.
- Call him and invite him to a late dinner in a romantic restaurant.
- Plan popcorn and a movie at home instead of dinner.
- If he has to work late, and it is appropriate to do so, show up with take-out Chinese and spend 20 minutes with him.
- Hold hands.
- Hug each other.
- Try not to nag him. If he won't fix things hire someone. It's not worth the stress on the marriage.
- Give up the TV once in a while and cuddle instead.
- If he gets home late, leave a cup of hot chocolate in the microwave with directions for heat up!
- If possible, make an effort be up with him at one end of the day. The early morning or late night hours can be an opportunity to chat, or hold hands, or just have a few minutes of peace together.
- Buy him new socks for no reason, or a funny pair of boxers and put them in his drawer with a note.
- Tell him something meaningful every week (you may be too busy or not see one another to make it happen every day),

- o "You are a wonderful husband"
- o "You are a great father"
- o "You are a kind and comforting human being"
- o "What would your patients do without your care?"
- o "Thank you for all you do for this family"

- Once in a while, leave a tiny gift and a note in the car so he finds it when he goes to work. It can be anything- a gift certificate for a cup of coffee, a new key chain, a cigar. It's not really the gift that matters- it's the gesture of love.

- If your man isn't one to talk about things- leave him a series of small notes for a week, each one telling him one reason that you fell in love with him.

- Give him a back rub.

- Get in the shower with him and wash his back.

- Rub his feet as an act of thoughtfulness.

- Reminisce about when you first met and fell in love. You may have to start, but he may join in as he travels back in time with you.

- Organize his dresser drawers so they are neat when he opens them and things are easy to find.

- Buy him a new toothbrush.

- Tell him "You look very handsome today."

- Tell him "Have I told you lately that I can't live without you?"

- Go to the bookstore together, or the sporting goods store, whatever he likes, and wander the aisles together.
- If mornings are hectic and you are getting the kids ready for school at the same time, send them to him to give him a kiss for no reason.
- While they are doing their homework, have them create a heart shaped note for him and put it in his car.
- Have them put tiny love notes in his coat pockets.

Tools For Him:

It is the simple gestures that keep a relationship alive, fresh and loving. It doesn't take a 2 week vacation to make your partner or spouse feel valued. These simple things do wonders to keep the love, and the communication, alive.

For example: when you are watching Gray's Anatomy together, snuggle up to her, and whisper: Babe, I love that you are a doctor, and that you can heal people.

She will hear: I love you, I love the fact you heal people, I know you are the real deal. Gray's Anatomy is only a dramatization of doctors, but we both still like to watch it.

Other simple gestures include:

- Buy her one piece of chocolate and leave it on her pillow.
- Buy her a gift certificate for a pedicure.

- Keep chilled wine in the refrigerator.
- Buy a new cup for her tea or coffee and leave it on the counter.
- Pick wildflowers and put them in a vase.
- Ask her "How are you today?"
- Ask, "How was your day?"
- Ask, "Yesterday you said you had a headache. Is it gone?"
- Call and leave a message on her voice mail telling her you love her.
- Make a lunch date with her in the middle of the week.
- Meet on a park bench with her favorite tea or coffee.
- Call her just to say you are thinking of her.
- Get a babysitter without her asking, and go on a movie date.
- Tell her she is beautiful.
- Say "I love you."
- In the small moments of the day, when passing in the house, grab her and hug her.
- Ask her "Have I told you lately that I appreciate everything you do?"
- Tell her she is a great mother.
- Take her away for an afternoon to walk along the beach, stroll through town, or get an ice cream cone.

- Call her hairdresser and buy an expensive jar of hair or skin care treatment that will be waiting for her at her next appointment.
- Buy aromatherapy soap and put it in the shower for her.
- Be kind.
- When you get up to go into another room, ask "Can I get anything for you?"
- Tell her she is beautiful. (Yes that is repeated from above. It's important!)
- Post your favorite picture of the two of you on the refrigerator as a surprise.
- Bring home take out when she least expects it.
- If you are home and she is working late, call her and tell her "Dinner is taken care of". You will be her hero.
- Put the dishes in the dishwasher to show you care. (Really!)
- Fluff her pillows before she goes to bed.
- Sit beside her on the couch while watching TV.
- Buy a card, any silly card, write a thoughtful note on it, and leave it in her purse.
- Turn off your laptops and tablets, the TV, the radio, your cell phones if possible, and talk to one another.
- If your schedules are impossibly hectic, find one common ½ hour that is free and make it a regular date for coffee. Put it on your calendar in red- it cannot be disrupted- with no exceptions.

10 SEX AND BURNOUT

"The best sex education for kids is when Daddy pats Mommy on the fanny when he comes home from work." William Masters

Why do I open this chapter with that quote? Because it captures the essence of what sex should be- joyous, intimate, happy and full of love. All of that is reflected in that simple action of patting "Mommy on the fanny". It is a light-hearted, affection gesture, and that is something we should all have in our lives. Burnout prevents that – all of that- but hopefully by reading this book, you will begin to discover the steps that will lead you out of the darkness of burnout. So, let's talk about sex and what happens to it when burnout becomes the third partner in the bedroom.

WeI have discussed at length what burnout does to the individual: creates low self-esteem, obsession with work resulting in long work hours, emotional exhaustion, depression, decline in family relationships, denial of self needs, and more. This list alone highlights the impact of burnout on one's sex life so let's examine it in a bit more detail.

Low self-esteem: It stands to reason that if you do not like yourself you are not going to think anyone else is attracted to, or wants you, even your spouse. This immediately affects the sexual dynamic.

Long work hours: Chances are you are not going to invite your spouse into your office for a sexual triste when you are concentrating on your work. When you are in any of the stages of burnout, the reason that you are working long hours is because you now believe that you are the only one who can do the job correctly and that if work long enough you will prove yourself indispensable. This certainly will not cause you to think it is time to have sex on your desk!

Emotional exhaustion: Burnout is burning you from the inside out. It has left you with little ability to feel compassion for your patients, no tolerance for your staff, and no desire to get involved with the lives of your loved ones. In other words, you are probably going to shut out your spouse because you don't have the emotional bandwidth to entertain a discussion on the day's events, problems at home or intimate talk between the sheets.

Depression: This most evil of emotional conditions has made your world a dark place. You believe you can do nothing right, no one likes you or approves of you; you feel helpless and useless. Where is the joy in life? Where in the midst of it all do you feel like sharing yourself with your partner or spouse and having sex? Making love is even more unlikely because it requires exposing oneself and making oneself vulnerable to the emotion.

Decline in family relationships: If you have excluded yourself from family relationships one of three things is happening;

1) You aren't talking to your spouse or partner much and so the warm-up to sex has no chance to occur.

2) You have shut down and your children no longer try to have conversations with you.

3) Your spouse or partner is so angry with you for alienating the family that the last thing he or she wants to do is have sex with you.

Denial of self needs: Let's face it; we were born to have sex. You knew that before you went to medical school. It is a basic, biological force in every human being. However, as you suffer from burnout, you lose touch with everything you need, including the need for intimacy and human touch.

It's a depressing list, isn't it? You can see how burnout has the power to gut the most intimate needs we have- sexual gratification, and intimacy with our partners and the human touch. And yet, when one searches the literature there is very, very little on the matter of burnout and sex. One can find many studies about depression and sex after surgery, cardiac arrest, violence, drug use, mental illness and any number of multiple diagnosis conditions. When it comes to burnout and sex, it is obvious that there remains a lot of work to be done to understand the syndrome in this context. This underscores our belief that the best physicians, scientists and psychologists need to put their efforts into the study and treatment of burnout syndrome in the medical community.

Given the lack of literature on the subject, I am going to extract my own conclusions by using the relationship that exists between depression and sex. Depression is a key component of burnout syndrome. Therefore, we are going to take the liberty of making the assumption that if burnout creates depression and depression impacts sex, then burnout impacts sex. We are not sex experts by any means, so to begin our discussion we are going to quote extensively from studies and literature that have examined the impact of depression on sexual activity and libido.

The study, "Sexual Dysfunction in Populations with Depression" was conducted in Switzerland. The study reported that, "There is (also) a broad consensus that the occurrence of sexual dysfunction is consistently higher in patients with depression than in the general population. The overall prevalence of sexual problems in patients with depression was approximately twice that of controls (50% vs. 24%)."

Another study on depression and sexual desire was conducted at the University of Missouri-Columbia School of Medicine and it too finds a direct correlation between depression and a lack of sexual activity. In their report, Robert L. Phillips, Jr., M.D., and

James R. Slaughter, M.D. included the following findings:

"In one study it was found that more than 70 percent of depressed patients had a loss of sexual interest when not taking medication, and they reported that the severity of this loss of interest was worse than the other symptoms of depression. In this same study, libido declined with increasing severity of psychological illness."

Drs. Phillips and Slaughter go on to say that the status of relationships has an impact on sexual relationships as well:

"It is important to assess the patient for psychological and interpersonal factors that commonly affect depression and sexual desire. These factors include stressful life events (loss of job or family trauma), life milestones (children leaving home) and ongoing relationship problems. Patients with major depressive disorder or bipolar disorder have an even higher prevalence of sexual dysfunction, including lowered libido, than the general population."

We also know that physicians suffering from burnout may begin to self-medicate with drugs or alcohol in an attempt to fill the internal void that they feel on a daily basis. This feeds into sexual problems as well:

"Alcohol and narcotics are known to decrease libido, arousal and orgasm. Because the use of alcohol and other drugs is more common in patients with psychological disorders, alcohol and drug abuse should be considered when investigating libido problems in patients with depression."

Outside of the purely clinical, scientific journals and research studies, there is ample evidence of depression and its impact. We are going to talk about how to improve your sex life, but before we do, we need to look further into the effect that depression has on relationships. It is important to do so. Why focus so much on depression? Because it lies at the heart of burnout. It feeds on itself and gathers strength by stealing from other parts of your life. Depression is like fingers of fog. Picture those nights when you have driven past a dark meadow and noticed the fog extending its fingers across the road, moving slowly, stealth-like until it covers your path. That is exactly how depression moves in your life; it moves slowly until it covers every inch of your daily life.

Psychologists, psychiatrists and therapists regularly treat patients who are suffering from this potentially disabling disease. Fortunately they share their knowledge, posting it online for general consumption. In the event that you or your spouse should begin to seek increased understanding of depression as part of the burnout you may be experiencing, you can begin the process from the privacy of your own home.

For example, Melissa Fritchle, LMFT, MA, is a therapist who works with patients whose depression is seriously affecting their sex life. She wrote an article called "Being Depressed Can Ruin a

Man's Sex Drive". Here we find many connections between the symptoms of burnout and the impact they can have on one's sex life. Her experience with her patients discovered a causal connection between depression, relationships, sex and more. If it were possible, we would insert "burnout" into her text because the syndrome is so deeply connected to the issues that she discusses.

"When people are asked why they have sex, the most common answers, for both men and women, are for pleasure and to feel connected to the other person. What happens when a person's sense of pleasure is critically dampened? Not only may motivation and drive for sexual activity go down, but so do fantasies about sex, which can strengthen one's libido. It is no surprise that many people with depression report decreased sex drives. Add to this the general sense of being overwhelmed, exhaustion, and difficulty functioning through daily activities that may be a part of depression and having sex may become another example in their life of 'going through the motions'."

And then we see the direct correlation, as her patient studies bring forward the issue of perfectionism, which, as we have discussed elsewhere in this book, is a key sign of burnout.

"Perfectionism/Pressure: When talking to people suffering from depression, what we often find is a very critical mind, a tendency to have high, often unrealistic, expectations and a pattern of focusing on the negative aspects of past experiences. Any sex therapist will tell you perfectionism is an enemy to sexual performance and satisfaction. Putting unrealistic expectations onto a sexual experience will led to pressure, stress, and difficulty being present for the fun of what is happening. This can lead to performance anxiety, erectile dysfunction, early ejaculation, and a lower libido. All of which can also lead to an increase in depression symptoms."

And then there is the danger zone:

"Some men with depression report turning to sexual behaviors that don't make them feel good in the big picture. Increased porn use may cause unrealistic expectations or disconnection or isolation from partners. Seeking out new partners may complicate or betray current relationship agreements. Feeling forced to have sex with their partner to relieve their pain may create pressure or resentment in that relationship. These men may feel like their sexuality slips into a compulsive behavior, driven by a need to escape negative feelings rather than a positive drive. Conflicted feelings about sexual behaviors can create a feedback loop that increase feelings of depression, leading to more drive to escape those feelings, and on it goes."

Depression is so insidious, that it doesn't stop once it has ruined your sex life, your ability to function daily and subtracted most of the joy from your life. No, depression keeps going, affecting the people around you. At home, depression significantly impacts your family because it creates "caregivers". Eventually, someone who loves you is going to become the point person in taking care of you.

Healthline.com posted an insightful article that discussed depression as a disease that creates caregivers. In the context of our discussion about burnout and sex, we can all understand that when you spend your days taking care of someone, that is not conducive to feeling sexually attracted to them. After all, the caregiver begins to feel emotional exhaustion just as the depressed person does.

"Depression is an illness that by its very nature undermines many of the aspects of a loving relationship that make it possible to continue the struggle when things become difficult. Relationships thrive on communication, for example, and a certain amount of give and take, but depression erodes both of these. Meaningful communication is often one of the first casualties of depression, and depressed people simply lose the energy to give or the will to take.

"People who are depressed are literally not themselves, and that makes it difficult for both parties to remain committed to working things out. People who are depressed are likely to lose interest in activities that both partners formerly enjoyed. They are likely to lose interest in sex, for example, and may find it difficult to sleep—or to get out of bed."

A recent study in the Journal of Psychophysiology, reported in

Women's Health online magazine, "surveyed over 300 couples about their marital stress—things like how often they felt let down by their partner or how often their spouse criticized them—and their symptoms of depression. Then, nine years later, they repeated those surveys with the same couples. They also asked participants to undergo emotional response testing, which basically involved measuring each person's frown muscles as they looked at a mix of negative, positive, and neutral photographs.

"The connections were startling: participants who reported the highest marital stress throughout the study also showed the most signs of depression. For instance, those with higher marital stress also smiled less at the positive photographs, an indication that they weren't able to fully enjoy positive experiences—a hallmark of depression.

"Worth noting here is that the study only showed correlation, not causation. That means that while it's absolutely possible (and makes some level of sense) that marital stress can make you feel depressed, it's also possible that suffering from depression and depression-related symptoms might also impact the amount of marital stress that you report feeling. Depression is a serious disease that can have a negative impact on every area of your life, including relationships."

Does feeling responsible for everything make you a bad sex partner?

Probably. First because it means that you are trying to handle everything yourself. Secondly the more responsibility you bear, the more your exhaustion increased. Thirdly, if you are bearing the weight of responsibility it means that you are not sharing it with your partner or spouse. The result is that there is less communication in the relationship, your spouse feels left out of your life, and intimacy declines.

The literature shows that "Sex under these conditions creates distance in the relationship or creates sexual dysfunction which drives an even deeper wedge into the relationship. This is especially true if a man is married to a woman must be wanted by her husband to have her sexuality validated.

Consequently, sex routinely becomes mechanical, unfeeling, and unfulfilling. Fortunately, anyone can break this vicious cycle and restore closeness, intimacy, and sexual flow in the relationship."

More Intellect- Less Sex

This subject would not be complete without calling attention to the fact that intellectuals have less sex than the less educated people. Many studies have shown that intellectuals, who have spent their lives exerting control, are the least likely to give up control for a pursuit such as sex. It is an activity that while immensely pleasurable, requires the antithesis of what an intellectual regularly seeks in life. Sex requires spontaneity, raw emotions, and leaving deep thought behind in order to engage in intense physical pleasure.

A study published in the Journal of Sexual Medicine called, "The Sexual Lives of Residents and Fellows in Graduate Medical Education Programs: A Single Institution Survey" set out to "explore the sexual behavior of (medical) residents and fellows in training and to determine the incidence of sexual dysfunction in this population.

Here I quote the study: "Main Outcome Measures. The validated survey instruments selected were the International Index of Erectile Function (IIEF), the Index of Premature Ejaculation (IPE), and the Self-Esteem and Relationship Quality (SEAR) survey for male residents, and the Female Sexual Function Index (FSFI) and the Index of Sex Life (ISL) for female residents. Results were compared with established normative data and validated cut-off scores that were available. Pearson correlation coefficient was used to assess for relationships between variables.

"Results: There were 180 responses (83 female, 97 male, mean age 29 years), for a response rate of 20%. Among men, 90%, 67%, and 98% were in a relationship, married, and heterosexual, respectively. Among women, the same numbers were 80%, 55%, and 96%, respectively. Based on validated cut-off scores for the IIEF and FSFI, 13% of men reported ED (3% reported mild ED, 4% reported moderate ED, and 6% reported severe ED) and 60% of women were classified as "at high risk" for sexual problems, with desire disorders the most prevalent and orgasmic disorders the second most prevalent. There were significant gender differences with respect to the associations between sexual and relationship problems."

An article in Medical Daily reiterated that "It's possible that students with high IQs aren't having much sex, resorting to sex toys as a means of achieving sexual gratification. This theory reinforces what researchers have said time and time again for years: people with higher IQs have less sex than everyone else."

Sociologist Rosemary Hopcroft discussed this theory in detail in a 2011 article published in Psychology Today. She said that the incidence of lower sexual activity in intellectuals is "a bit dismaying".

Psychology Today said that people who have attended institutions of higher learning have sex less frequently and have fewer sexual partners than those who do not, reporting that Hopcroft's studies reaffirmed this theory, "Her contentions were confirmed by a joint sex survey by MIT and Wellesley College that found that a high IQ can delay sexual activity into early adulthood.

"According to a 2007 article entitled "Intercourse and

Intelligence," 80 percent of U.S. males and 75 percent of U.S. women have had sex by the age of 19. Compare that to 56 percent of Princeton undergraduates, 59 percent of Harvard undergraduates and 51 percent of MIT undergraduates who report having had sexual intercourse. What's more, only 65 percent of MIT graduate students have had sex."

While this remains a theory, scientific studies continue to find that it remains true. Again we refer to studies reported in Psychology Today.

"The latest National Survey of Family Growth shows that, for example, men with college degrees are half as likely to have had four or more partners in the last year as men with a high school education alone. (Or at least, they're half as likely to admit it, points out Anjani Chandra, a health scientist and demographer at the Centers for Disease Control.)

Why? "It's hard to pick apart," Chandra says. But the sexual habits of teens might offer a clue. Carolyn Halpern, a professor at the UNC School of Public Health, found a high concentration of teen virgins at the top of the intelligence scale. She thinks the smartest kids might hold off on sex because they're thinking through its potential consequences.

In her studies Hopcroft wondered about the causes of reduced sexual activity among intellectuals; "Smart people having less sex and starting to have sex later in life can be attributable to any number of things. People with higher IQs may take into consideration the negative consequences of risky sexual behavior more than their peers of average intelligence. They could also just be too busy studying and working to find time for sexual relationships with others. Or they could be lacking in good looks."

However, the Psychology Today report says researchers conducting many of the studies on this issue have accounted for these variables, eliminating them from the "reduced sexual activity" equation: "Other researchers analyzing the link between sex and intelligence, control for attractiveness, personal grooming, and affability, and the observed effect still holds. It might be a question of priorities: "Pursuing education takes up a lot of time," Chandra says.

When it comes to understanding why intellectual adults have less sex, researchers turn to Life History Theory, which examines how species have evolved different reproductive strategies to survive, for a possible explanation. "People with high executive functioning—in judgment, decision-making, and impulse control—usually have what's called a slow life history strategy," notes Aurelio José Figueredo, an evolutionary psychologist at the University of Arizona. "They tend to have fewer partners and less sex but more resources (such as money and status) to invest in potential offspring."

The next part of this discussion may seem like a detour, but it is actually one of the most enlightening findings of our cumulative research. Why? Because this idea applies to all of us, of all ages, in this technological age. It goes to the heart and tenor of many relationships today and serves as a warning that if we are not careful, our phones may replace our humanity. It is a red flag calling attention to the fact that if we do not teach our children the skills needed for healthy intimacy, then how are they to have healthy intimate relationships as adults?

Marty Klein, PhD, author, certified sex therapist, and licensed marriage and family therapist for 30 years, posted this blog on Psychology Today's online "Sexual Intelligence" column. With thanks we reprint this excerpt to serve as a guidepost for all of us:

"It appears that many young men and women don't entirely recognize each other as fellow beings. They're just not that curious about each other, and so they don't see face-to-face, personal communication as a wonderful opportunity. Rather than being a familiar, foundational activity, face-to-face talking is an intrusion into what really matters—checking your iPhone.

"And that's exactly what we need to be concerned about: we've stopped teaching our children how to communicate face-to-face with other human beings. We take children too young to have fully learned how to participate in relationships, give them the most advanced technology for impersonal, asynchronous 'communication' in the history of the world, and let them use these devices at the dinner table, while being driven to school, and any other time they have to interface with adults—people who might actually help them learn something about relationships. And kids naturally use them with each other, too—an average of 93 times per day.

"What happens? When the time comes, they have little idea how to date, court, or create one-on-one, face-to-face relationships. They haven't learned how to ask a real person real questions—watching that person's face as they listen to the answer. They've never experienced the risk of reaching out to take someone's hand—and watched that person's face as they agreed or declined.

"If we don't teach children to relate, don't demand that they engage, and give them the means for endless solitary entertainment, they cannot and will not learn to relate in a deep way.

"Historically, most people have had their marriages arranged for them, and they've managed well enough. But they rarely thought they were in love, and they generally weren't pursuing some ideal of 'intimacy', which people today claim they desire. In contrast, today's young people (eventually) want to fall in love, and say they (eventually) want intimacy. You need skills for that. And today's young people simply aren't learning those skills. It's easy to have sex. It's way harder to have a relationship in which you have sex.

"Now please don't blame porn. It's true--and ridiculous--that some men expect women to be porn stars, and some women are trying to compete with porn actresses, but that's not the point. If porn now provides a template for the non-relationships that young men (and increasingly young women) value, we have to ask why such a template looks attractive. The answer is that too many young people have nothing more intimate to compare it to. Young people aren't learning to embrace anyone—because they're not learning to want to embrace anyone.

"So moms and dads, don't give your kids smartphones and unlimited digital access until they're at least 40 years old.

'OK, here's Plan B: demand that your kids learn how to interact with actual people. You, of course, will have to be some of those actual people. Those phones your kids use are your phones, not theirs, so establish phone-free hours in their lives (including between bed-time and breakfast, when kids exchange millions of text messages)."

Let's adopt these ideas as intellectuals. Let's be ever mindful of the importance of face-to-face connection. Let's keep this information present as we consider the theories we have discussed on why intellectuals have less sex.

Sexual activity is important in your life

I have already discussed how sex can release endorphins that help to fight the depression that is part of burnout syndrome. Sex can make you feel that you are important to someone, raise your self-esteem because you feel desired, and release stress. All of these are important in the fight to reduce the symptoms of burnout syndrome. That gives us several explanations of why intellectuals have less sex. However, it does not dismiss the importance of sexual activity in your life. We have already discussed how sex can release endorphins that help to fight the depression that is part of burnout syndrome. Sex can make you feel that you are important to someone, raise your self-esteem because you feel desired, and release stress. All of these are important in the fight to reduce the symptoms of burnout syndrome.

So how are you supposed to increase your sex life if you are burned out? What are you supposed to do if you don't have the energy to eat, you can't sleep, you feel as though you are unattractive, and yet we are telling you that more sex is good?

Here are some suggestions on how to rev up your relationships in the bedroom. Consider it ways to sex up your sex life.

Is there any good news?

Yes there is, so let's get to it. It is possible to improve your sex life, revive intimacy and love fully and actively again. If you are suffering from burnout it is going to take some work because you are going to have to access positive emotions that by now may be deeply buried. That is where you have to begin because as Mae

West said, "Sex is emotion in motion."

It takes a connection to have great sex (and not just a physical one!).

Okay, that's easy to understand, but how does one begin to renew a connection with one's lover? What exactly is great sex?

To answer that I went directly to the readers of about.com's sexuality forum. In response to the article, "What is Great Sex, Readers Respond", one reader posted, "Great sex, for me, happens when you completely give all of yourself to your partner, mind and body, and try to fulfill their desires of pleasure. You have to be kind of selfless. And then with trust and selflessness, you exchange great pleasure."

That is both a great definition of sex, and the reason that sex can be so problematic while suffering from burnout syndrome. Just look at some of the words the reader used: "selfless", "trust", "give all of yourself". These are the antithesis of what burnout allows you to feel. Burnout removes trust, makes you selfish and self-centered. You give all of yourself, but to your job, not to your loved ones. The very things that create intimacy, close relationships, honest marriages and great sex are the same things that are stripped away due to burnout. However, this also gives you a starting point. Choose one and get to work on it. If you are being selfish by working all the time, purposely leaving no time for family relationships, start small. Select one night for a special dinner with your spouse or partner. Keep the "appointment" and don't be late. Leave your cell phone, pager, and tablet in the car. Pay attention, close attention to him or her during dinner. If you can achieve this for just one or two hours, you have successfully made your first step toward selflessness.

For women, great sex is about relationships

That's not to say there aren't many women who just want sex because it feels good. There are. However, what we are talking about here is sex in a relationship, with the person you go home to every night, or who shares a special place in your life. Mechanical sex does not include a connection or bond with your partner. If you are suffering from burnout, you need a connection and you need intimacy. You need the human touch because it is soothing and reassuring. It makes you feel valued and wanted; all the emotions that burnout is stripping from you.

Great sex for women includes intimacy, trust and touching

Psychologist and author Gina Ogden, Ph.D. wrote the book, "Women Who Love Sex". In it she describes her interviews with many women regarding sex and what great sex means to them. She says that they "described peak sexual experiences as coming from stimulation all over their bodies--not just from their genitals--including fingers, toes, hips, lips, neck, and earlobes.

Obviously, arousal and satisfaction evolve not only from receiving sexual energy, but also from the joy of stimulating one's partner. Sex, then, is a commitment of give and take."

Anthony Fiore, Ph.D., reported on Dr. Ogden's findings, pointing out an interesting redefinition of "safe sex". "The women Dr. Ogden studied have their own concepts of safe sex, essential to experiencing sexual pleasure and ecstasy. This kind of safe sex does not relate to preventing STDs or pregnancy; it relates, instead, to emotional and spiritual safety. Such safety is crucial for sexual closeness. Most of the women insisted that warm, loving connections with themselves and with their partners were essential to and inseparable from the experience of sexual ecstasy.

When people feel deeply close while merely holding hands, they are having sex. When people display caring for each other through hugs, caresses, and kissing, they are also having sex. When connecting people in a crowded room wink at each other in their own secret way, they are communicating sex to each other; such non-contact sex can be excitedly arousing and emotionally fulfilling. And, of course, during sexual union when the sky seems to open so a lightning bolt can strike the couple--while fireworks ignite and the earth stops spinning-- this is sex, too."

Do men also need this connection to enjoy sex? Dr. Fiore says he believes the answer is "Yes and no. Men need sex and men need emotional connection, but many men don't necessarily need to put the two together!"

Great sex requires communication

This is where it gets a bit tricky. When you are suffering from burnout, the last thing you want to do is open an intimate conversation with your partner. However, without communication your sex life is not going to get back on track. Communication is a key to intimacy. It is a key to being attracted to one another, at least for the long term. The problem is that communication requires opening ourselves to one another. After all, you aren't going to talk about the weather to feel sexually attracted to each other! No, you are going to have to open yourself, share part of yourself to open the lines of communication. If you are suffering from burnout, exposing part of your inner self to your partner is going to be frightening, if not impossible. Let's talk about it to find a way to take the first step toward opening yourself to intimate communication with your loved one.

Cory Silverberg is a sexuality expert who writes for about.com. His ground rules for sexual communication provide a constructive outline for partners who want to move from isolation to intimacy. Cory suggests, "You can pick and choose from these ideas, or use them as a launch pad to develop whatever rules feel right for everyone involved.

Time to Check In and Check Out

If you start a conversation when you're exhausted or angry about something else that happened that day, you'll bring those things into the conversation with you. One way to deal with this inevitability is to "check in" at the beginning of the conversation; spend a minute sharing something about your day and how you're feeling so you know what you're each coming to the conversation with. Do the same at the end of the conversation to say how you felt it went (but don't use that as a way to keep the conversation going after you've agree to end it). It's a nice idea to end each conversation sharing at least one positive thing that came out of it.

Define Safety for Yourselves and to Each Other

No one can be expected to communicate honestly and openly unless they feel safe. Make a list for yourself about what you need to feel safe and then share that list with your partner. Feeling safe might be about language that you use, or where you have the conversation. It might be agreeing to no yelling, or that neither of you will storm out of the room. If you can agree on things from your lists those can become part of the ground rules.

Respecting Differences in Sexual Interests

If the conversation you want to have is about sharing sexual fantasies or trying a new sexual activity together, everyone needs to agree not to belittle, shame, or otherwise laugh at their partner's sexual interests. This doesn't mean you have to like them or act them out. But if your partner takes the risk of exposing a sexual desire, you need to consider that kind of sharing a compliment and be respectful, even if you want nothing to do with the actual proposal.

Attend Without Interrupting

This is one the hardest ground rules to follow, but also one of the most important ones. You need to engage and attend to what your partner is telling you without interrupting. If you're interrupting and talking over each other, neither of you will ever feel heard. Agree to not interrupt and know that you'll both slip up, but when you do you'll apologize and try harder to pay attention and wait until your partner is finished before responding.

Bring a Sense of Goodwill to the Conversation

Hopefully it's true of your relationship that neither you nor your partner are trying to intentionally hurt the other or be mean to the other. If you believe this is true, try to remember it even when you're getting into it with each other. If you find yourself attacking (either in what you're saying or how you are saying it) remember this ground rule and back off a bit.

Make 'I' Statements

A basic rule of good communication is to avoid telling the other person how they feel or what they think (in reality, you have no idea). What you can do is communicate about yourself and your own feelings. And a simple way to do this is try to start sentences with "I", as in "I feel like this when you do that".

Respect Differences in Values and Feelings

Relationships require a lot of compromise, but that doesn't mean we don't get to have our own thoughts, values and feelings. Show each other enough respect to allow for differences without forcing either person to concede their beliefs. In the end, everyone has to compromise, but in the beginning everyone should be feel as if their perspective was acknowledged.

Be Specific, Ask Questions

Try to be as specific as you can be and avoid making sweeping general statements (e.g. "you always do this" "I can never do that"). If you find your partner making vague or general statements ask for clarification and ask questions to try and help both of you get a clearer idea of what specifically is the problem.

Anyone Can Call Time-Out at Any Time

For a conversation to feel safe, everyone needs to feel like they can leave at any point. This doesn't make it OK to storm out while your partner is in the middle of a sentence, but agree that either of you, at any point, can ask for a time out, or to end the conversation, as long as you also agree to pick it up at a later point.

Agree on Confidentiality

Everyone needs to feel like what they say in a private conversation stays private. You'll have to agree on the limits of that (is it OK to talk to a best friend? A brother or sister?) but whatever restrictions you put on it, you have to respect those and not break confidentiality."

Spice Up Your Sex – It's good for you!

"Sexual energy is one of our most powerful energies for creating health," says Christiane Northrup, M.D., author of Women's Bodies, Women's Wisdom. "Through the intimate connection with another, our stress hormones lower and our serotonin shoots through the roof."

What else do you need to know? Sex can make you feel better!

We're all adults here, so let's talk about making your sex life an exciting place to be. Let's put together a Sex Wish List that the two of you can share. Let's make it wild and exciting. Get out the whipped cream, stock up on batteries, find some satin sheets and let's get imaginative. We're going to explore different types of sex and the ways to get there. Open your mind, it's time to have great sex with your partner.

Sexy sex for free:

Remember what we wrote about earlier? Here's what women want that won't cost men a dime:

Peak sexual experiences from stimulation all over their bodies--not just from their genitals--including fingers, toes, hips, lips, neck, and earlobes.

Emotional and spiritual safety. Women insist that warm, loving connections with their partners are essential and inseparable from the experience of sexual ecstasy.

When connecting people in a crowded room wink at each other in their own secret way, they are communicating sex to each other; such non-contact sex can be excitedly arousing and emotionally fulfilling.

Sex in the morning…

Morning sex is not only better for your health and overall mood, but men, you'll last longer and finish stronger. Testosterone levels peak overnight, so in the morning, most men are ready to go, Harry Fisch, MD, author of Size Matters told Cosmopolitan. Between being well-rested and the high testosterone levels, men will have more energy and last longer during morning romps between the sheets.

Sex in the evening…

Think about bringing the romance back into your love making. Don't just jump in and make it another mechanical 10 minute interlude. Take your time. Touch each other. Be intimate. Think about making love with each other instead of "having sex". Talk to each other. You can talk dirty, but if you want to be romantic and intimate, speak softly and ask sexy questions.

- What makes your skin smell so good?
- Why are your eyes such a beautiful blue/brown/green/grey, etc.
- When I undressed you for the first time, do you know what I was thinking?
- Do you remember when we made love in the (fill in the place)?
- Do you know that you still make my heart race when you kiss me?

Sex in the summertime…

Cosmopolitan magazine asked its readers to tell them about their favorite experience having sex outdoors. Why not? We're not talking about having sex in the middle of the park! We are talking about thinking about sex in a new way to bring excitement and enjoyment back into your sex life and your relationship. Here is what some of the Cosmo readers had to say about their own experiences enjoying sex in the great outdoors:

"On a camping trip, we decided to take a midnight walk in the pouring rain and make out in the nearby forest. There's something about the rain that makes the sex so much better, getting soaking wet together, and then slowly undressing each other." —Katie E.

"I once did it behind a waterfall on the rocks. It was really romantic." —Mohsin S.

"We did it under the stars on a summer night in a field. It was chilly for the summer, so we had to work extra hard to keep ourselves warm. He was wearing glowsticks around his neck, so I got to see his sexy expressions." —Tonya D.

Let's play nurse…

Ok, you already have access to a white physician's coat, and a stethoscope, bring them home! You have the props, use them in role play. Role-playing might be on her "must try" list of sexual fantasies. It might feel ridiculous to you at first, you may not even want to bring your work home. But if you are going to try role play, why not start with something that feels familiar?

Advice for men- Sometimes it's the simple things

The website, askmen.com is worth a visit. It talks about many issues that arise in the bedroom with simple ideas and short lists. If you and your partner are exhausted, if you relationship is strained because one or both of you is suffering from burnout, you need to begin the process of revving up your sex life with simple steps. We think the article "5 Simple Moves to Boost Her Desire" is a primer to be followed, so with thanks to askmen.com, we are going to quote them here:

1- Place her arms behind her head

This is an absolutely fantastic (and very hot) move. Typical results include a very horny woman writhing beneath you, begging for more. Every woman, no matter how dominant, enjoys it when her man takes charge. This move makes the most of that fact and serves as an excellent bridge between foreplay and sex. As you slide over her body, take one of her wrists in your hand, slowly raise it over her head, and push it back toward the pillow. If she doesn't have strong objections, repeat the process with her other arm. Your grasp should remain at her wrists and your grip should be firm, but not painful... There's always the chance this will unnerve her more than it turns her on. If she's been abused in the past, this may not be enjoyable for her, though that certainly isn't a given. Pay close attention and you'll be able to gauge her comfort level and adjust your efforts (or discontinue them) accordingly. The best way to determine this is to simply ask if she likes it — in your sexiest voice, of course.

Best position for this move: Placing her arms behind her head during the missionary, or some variation, will put the icing on an otherwise boring cake.

2- Slip your hands into her hair

An under-utilized secret weapon, this one turns even the coldest of fish to mush in a relatively short time. No matter the length of her locks, having a man's hands in her hair can definitely result in wet knickers. Always start at the nape of the neck, as this area tends to be extremely sensitive. Gently trace the hairline and work your way upward into her hair; apply gentle pressure to the scalp as you delve into her tresses. It certainly will help, but you don't need to kiss her while doing this. And if you really want to spice it up, give her locks a gentle (but firm) tug. If you do, be sure to grasp a handful, and do so from the root — anything else could result in something unexpectedly painful for her.

Best position for this move: The beauty of this little number is its diversity. If you're already in bed, this can be used continuously and at any time. Just chilling on the sofa? Slide a little closer and see how quickly this turns her on. Kissing her goodnight on the doorstep? Try this baby out and you just might be invited up for a nightcap.

3- Be vocal in response to her efforts

For a woman, there's something very sexy about hearing a man groan with lust. The next time she's performing oral sex on you, let her hear what you're feeling. It'll boost her ego and give her the confidence to really let herself go. The sound of your heavy breathing can do wonderful things, as well. Just let her know you love what she's doing.

Best position for this move: Obviously, you can receive oral sex in a variety of positions. The best position for this scenario is one in which you can easily caress her face or hair. Touching her as she goes down on you will make her feel more secure, bolstering her confidence even further.

4- <u>Sweet talk her</u>

A well-chosen phrase spoken at the right time makes a woman feel like you want her, and not just her body. This is crucial for sex, as women want (and need) to feel a deeper connection. Because the average man doesn't say much during sex, your efforts to do so will give you an automatic edge. You might think that you need to recite Shakespeare or use a Barry White voice, but all you need is a whisper — really. What should you say? That's the easy part. Women will never, ever tire of hearing romantic phrases, as long as they sound genuine. "You're beautiful"; "I love your breasts"; "I love your body"; "Your skin is so soft"; and "I love you" are all simple, sweet little nothings designed to make her feel more in tune with you. Also, try not to exaggerate too much. Tell her she's beautiful. Tell her she's gorgeous. But don't tell her she's hotter than Heidi Klum unless she really is — you don't want her to feel patronized.

Best position for this move: Anytime, anyplace, anywhere. There isn't a bad time to compliment your woman. There just isn't.

5- Pay attention to her entire body

Few things are sexier than knowing someone can't keep their hands off of you. The single most important factor here is pace, so take your time to explore, caress and tease. Use your fingers, lips or the palms of your hands to trace the outline of her body, caress her face or gently massage her thighs as you wrap them around your waist. You can also run your fingertips over her lips, kiss her lightly on the cheek or slide your hands around her waist and squeeze gently. These little things will help a woman to feel close to you during sex and improve it exponentially. Keep your touch soft and smooth and she'll be purring in no time.

Best position for this move: Again, there isn't a wrong time to utilize this one. Indeed, you can, and should, make use of it as often as possible. And, if you're a man who has never done this in the past, it will be appreciated from the first try.

Practice makes perfect.

If you find any of these moves embarrassing, don't worry, you're not alone. Take comfort in knowing you really can't mess them up. Take them one at a time and don't worry about getting it perfect. The average woman will be thrilled with even a partial effort. As you explore her reactions, you'll be able to develop your own style and it'll be second nature before you know it. Sure, you can ignore these moves and keep on with better-than-average sex, but if you decide to try your hand at mind-blowing, hotter-than-hot sex, you're going to need a deeper connection with your partner — and these moves will help you get there."

Advice for women: Men want you to understand their needs.

For this we turn to WebMD with advice that will help women to understand what their man wants, and needs, to have a healthy sex life.

"OK, so maybe this one is no secret. Most men under age 60 think about sex at least once a day, compared with only a quarter of women. And that's not all. Men fantasize about sex nearly twice as often as women do, and their fantasies are much more varied. They also think more about casual sex than women do. But thinking is not the same as doing.

Men Find Sex Significant

It's a myth that most men think sex is just sex. For many, sex is a very important act between two committed people. And just like most women, men find sexual intimacy to be most satisfying within a committed relationship. One reason is that long-term partners know how to please one another better than strangers do.

He Likes It When You Initiate Sex

Most guys feel as though they're the ones who always initiate sex. But they also like to be pursued and wish their partner would take the lead more often. Don't be shy about letting your guy know you're in the mood. Initiating sex some of the time may lead to a higher level of satisfaction for both of you.

Guys Aren't Always Up for Sex

Men, much to many women's surprise, aren't always in the mood for sex. Just like women, men are often stressed by the demands of work, family, and paying the bills. And stress is a big libido crusher. When a guy says, "not tonight," it doesn't mean he's lost interest in you. He just means he doesn't want to have sex right then.

Men Like Pleasing Their Partner

Your pleasure is important to your man. But he won't know what you want unless you tell him. Too many women feel uncomfortable talking about what they like and don't like. If you can tell him clearly in a way that doesn't bruise his ego, he'll listen. Because he knows he'll feel good if you feel good.

Guys Get Performance Anxiety

Most men get performance anxiety on occasion, especially as they age. Your guy may worry about his body, technique, and stamina. If you can help him learn to relax and stay focused on the pleasures of the moment, sex will become less stressful.

Maybe it's time to take a walk on the wild side

Sex between two consenting adults can be as wild and spicy as you like. Toys and sex aides abound on the internet and even arrive in unmarked brown paper boxes. The neighbors will never know what you are up to (unless they buy the same toys!) and you can liven up your sex life without ever walking into an adult sex store. That's probably a good thing given the fact that you don't want to bump into one of your patients there! Start with scented oils and give each other a massage. There are a lot to choose from, including heated and flavored massage oils. Then you can move into using other toys to pleasure one another. Sex releases endorphins that help to fight depression. If you need a reason to have more sex- now you have one.

Sex after 50

Is there sex after 50? Yes, and lots of it.

1. You just have to get creative and adjust to what your 50 year old body wants to do- and it's not what your 25 year old body wanted to do.
2. You may not be able to pursue the sexual positions you could 25 years ago.

3. You may need more time to get aroused. But isn't that a good thing? Now you are older, you have probably mellowed a bit, so why not be more romantic as well?

4. Foreplay can be a romantic dinner, an erotic movie, or massaging one another.

The well-known author of passages, Gail Sheehy, wrote a book called "Sex and the Seasoned Woman- Pursuing the Passionate Life". The synopsis of her book says that women over 50 are ready, and willing, for sex and sexual adventure. "Boomer generation women in midlife are open to sex, love, dating, new dreams, exploring spirituality, and revitalizing their marriages as never before. This is a new universe of passionate, liberated women–married and single–who are unwilling to settle for the stereotypical roles of middle age and are now realizing they don't have to. As life spans grow longer and as societal constraints continue to loosen, older women–once free of the exhausting demands of young children, needy husbands, and demanding careers–find themselves ready to pursue the passionate life. They embrace their "second adulthood" as a period of reawakening."

AARP says that for men, sex in your 50's is the good news. This is a time when "men and women are more in sync. In their 20s and 30s, men become aroused more quickly than women, and many younger women complain: "He's all finished before I even feel aroused." But older men take longer to feel turned on. The transition to slower arousal can be disconcerting, but it means that the sexual discord of youth can evolve into new sexual harmony. 'Compared with young lovers, older couples are more sexually in sync,' says Dr. Richard Sprott, a developmental psychologist. 'Couples who appreciate this can enjoy more fulfilling sex at 65 than they had at 25 — even without erection and intercourse.'"

The great thing about sex after 50 is that now you can explore, experiment and find new pleasure together. Be creative. It will be good for you. Great sex with your partner will reassure you that you are loved. The physical contact will calm and soothe you. The time spent away from the demands of the world will reduce your stress and the endorphins released during sex will help your depression. All we really have in this world are the people we love. If you are suffering from burnout, loving is one of your best treatments, so use this chapter as a guide and get busy!

Resources and References:

18 Secrets Guys Wish You Knew http://**www.webmd.com**/sex-relationships/ss/slideshow-secrets-guys-wish-you-knew Reviewed by Nivin Todd, MD, FACOG on April 10, 2014

http://**www.aarp.org**/relationships/love-sex/info-10-2010/how_sex_changes_for_men_after_50.2.html
How Sex Changes for Men After 50- It's not the same as it used to be — and that can be a good thing
By: Michael Castleman, from: AARP, October 12, 2010

http://**www.askmen.com**/dating/love_tip_300/358_love_tip.html 5 Simple Moves To Boost Her Desire by Isabella Snow

http://**www.cosmopolitan.com**/sex-love/advice/g2039/best-outdoor-sex/?slide=2

http://**gailsheehy.com**/books/sex-and-the-seasoned-woman/overview/

http://**www.askmen.com**/dating/heidi_200/214_dating_girl.html

http://**www.businessinsider.com**/10-ways-to-improve-your-sex-life-2012-9?op=1#ixzz3VhkBEt2a

http://**www.womenshealthmag.com**/sex-and-relationships/ultimate-sex

Sexual Dysfunction, Depression, and the
Impact of Antidepressants
Sidney H. Kennedy, MD, FRCPC*Þ and Sakina Rizvi, HBSc*þ
http://**www.researchgate.net**/publication/26279323_Sexual_dysfunction_depression_and_the_impact_of_antidepressants

Depression and Relationships
http://**www.healthline.com**/health/depression/relationships#1
Written by Dale Kiefer | Published on March 29, 2012
Medically Reviewed by George Krucik, MD

http://**www.pbs.org**/thisemotionallife/blogs/being-depressed-can-ruin-mans-sex-drive

http://www.aafp.org/afp/2000/0815/p782.html   Depression and Sexual Desire
ROBERT L. PHILLIPS, JR., M.D., and JAMES R. SLAUGHTER, M.D., University of Missouri–
Columbia School of Medicine, Columbia, Missouri
American Family Physician. 2000 Aug 15;62(4):782-786.

http://www.womenshealthmag.com/sex-and-relationships/marriage-stress-and-depression
WOMEN'S HEALTH ONLINE MAGAZINE
Study: Marital Stress Is Linked to Symptoms of Depression
Here's how to fix it before it's too late
PUBLISHED: APRIL 28, 2014 | BY ARIELLE PARDES

Readers Respond: What Is Great Sex?
By Cory Silverberg   http://sexuality.about.com/u/ua/sexinformation/what_is_great_sex.htm

http://www.healthyplace.com/sex/good-sex/what-makes-for-good-sex/
Healthy Place America's Mental Health Channel- Sex-Sexuality Community, What Makes for Good
Sex?
Written by Anthony Fiore, Ph.D

http://sexuality.about.com/od/improvingsexcommunication/a/ground_rules.htm
Sexual Communication Ground Rules
Establishing Rules of Communication for Talking about Sex with a Partner
 By Cory Silverberg
Sexuality Expert

Read more: http://www.care2.com/greenliving/tantric-sex-for-beginners-4-easy-
tips.html#ixzz3Vhi1CAHa

http://www.todays-intimate-couple.com/senior-sex.html

11 IMMEDIATE ACTION PLAN FOR BURNOUT SYNDROME

If you are suffering from burnout syndrome, it is important to start with these interventions as soon as possible. Once you have begun to work on these issues and feel you are making some progress, then you can consider tackling some of the more complex issues of burnout.

Rapid action items:

1- Improve your sleep cycle.
2- Increase your total hours of sleep per week, and make an extra effort to regularly catch up on missing sleep due to the call schedule or family responsibilities.
3- Take your time getting ready in the morning because leaving the house already stressed achieves nothing.
4- Eat light, healthy meals frequently to avoid fluctuations in blood sugar. Avoid overeating and fatty food, but at the same time make sure to eat foods you like in moderation. Avoid being on diets to lose weight or gain muscle during this acute intervention period.

5- Take a mental break during your work day. This is best accomplished by taking a walk. If this is not possible, carve out a bit of uninterrupted time for yourself. Just 10 or 15 minutes of listening to music or using a mindless relaxation mobile app will serve the purpose. Avoid checking e-mails or completing any other work tasks during this time.

6- If after taking this break you find yourself getting irritated by patients, or you become suddenly short tempered with your staff, you will have to give yourself another 5-10 minutes of mental rest. DO NOT push through your irritation. This is one of the signs you need to pay attention to and you are in the rapid action phase of recovery.

Semi-Rapid action items:

Identify items in your daily life that bring you negative energy (feeling down), and those that bring you positive energy (feeling good). Try to shift the balance so that there are more positive energy sources in your daily life than negative. This may require taking a half-day off each week, or doing the unthinkable by completing your notes on the weekend in order to free some time during the week. BEWARE: your burned out brain is going to tell you that you don't have to do this, that you can take an afternoon off next week. You cannot delay. In order to get well you need to follow these steps. If you have to, print this list and check off the steps you take each day. It is going to take time for you to develop new habits that will help you recover from burnout. You are going to have to ignore your brain for a while!

Examples of items with negative energy:

Work related:

I- Paper work

II- Complex patients or second opinions

III- Feeling isolated in solo practice, or isolated due to the simple fact that all of your colleagues have very busy schedules.

IV- Being on call

V- Taking extra shifts

VI- Not enough time for patient encounters.

Personal life related:

I- Problems with children at school

II- Shopping for groceries

III- Honey-do's

IV- A relative with Alzheimer's or other chronic, long-term disease

V- An unhappy marriage

VI- An insensitive, nagging, unhappy spouse

VII- Caregiving for sick or aging relatives

Examples of items with positive energy:

Work related:

I-   Interaction with colleagues

II-   Grateful patients

III-   Successful patient/family conference

IV-   Making a difficult diagnosis that may result in successful treatment

V-   Supportive, productive staff

VI-   Watching patients get well and thrive under your care

VII-   Watching your practice grow

Personal life related:

I-   Playing with your children

II-   Going out to dinner with friends

III-   Seeing a movie in your favorite genre- action, romance, film noir, etc.

IV-   Listening to music

V-   Reading a book by your favorite author

VI-   Cuddling with your partner

VII-   Petting your dog or cat

VIII-   Taking a nap

IX-   Sitting outside in the sun

Non-Rapid Action Items:

To accomplish these items successfully, you are going to have to invest more time in the organization and prioritization of daily activities. On average, it has been shown that successfully prioritizing your day and streamlining work can actually free up to one hour of time. Here are some tips on how do to that:

I-   Respond to your e-mails as you open them. Do not leave e-mails to address later. The same principal applies to opening the mail; do it in one setting and do not "postpone" dealing with certain items till later on, they will only accumulate.

II-   Start an exercise program. You can take a walk during lunch time, a walk after work, or go to the gym 2-3 times a week. You must start slowly and increase your activity gradually. During the rapid action phase of recovery, your goal is not fitness. Your goal is taking time away from work to do something that is good for you, and good for your brain. Avoid listening to medical material while working out. You will negate all the benefits of the exercise.

III-   If you are already a runner, swimmer, or bicyclist, it is very important to add variety to your work. Find a way to include time at the gym, or some other varied workout so that you will have the opportunity to meet new people.

IV- If you are an accomplished athlete and obsessed with your training and fitness routine, consider that this could be one more early warning sign of burnout syndrome. Obsession with your training could be an effort to fill the void left by dissatisfaction with your work, a void generated by burnout syndrome. As an advanced athlete, you might consider breaking the cycle of your training addiction by giving some of that scheduled time to coaching lower level athletes and/or school teams. You should definitely consider getting involved in team sports on a fun, non-competitive level. Many gyms have a schedule of pick-up teams in any number of sports, like basketball or tennis. This is NOT the time to master a new sport! It is a time to have fun without the goal of winning the race. I realize this is potentially a very difficult task for the accomplished athlete. Breaking your training routine will involve a significant amount of personnel struggle. In fact, you may find that it is too difficult to give up and return to your rigorous workout. Don't give up your efforts to change quickly. Remember, this is a program, a remedy to help you heal. It is not going to be easy. This is a time to relax and have fun. It is not a time to excel in athletic pursuits.

V-   As I mentioned at the beginning of this section, it is important that you begin to practice the daily prioritization of tasks in order to organize your time. As you get better at this, you will notice the amount of time that is freeing up in increasing. Eventually, you may find that you have an extra hour of time each day. Here is what we want you to do with that hour- nothing. That's right. For one hour we want you to do absolutely nothing. I fully realize that this goes against everything you have ever practiced. In fact, it probably goes against your personality, your work ethic and several other values that you hold dear. Here is what you have to remember: mastering the art of relaxation is going to recharge you, reenergize you, reorder your thoughts, sort out your worries, and improve your health. As the guilt recedes, this may become your favorite hour of the day. Throughout your many years of schooling and the grueling hours of your career, you have mastered the art of utilizing every second for some productive purpose. Right now, your highest and most productive purpose is to heal yourself and recover from burnout. Now is the time to learn the most difficult task of all- relaxation. It is essential that you learn to invest one hour a day in the rejuvenation of your brain - doing nothing - and not feeling guilty about it.

VI-   If you are a male physician you may find this recommendation one of the hardest to accomplish: take a warm bath once a week, get a neck message once every 2 weeks, and get a facial once a month. Do not freak out now, this is only a temporary remedy for the male physician. And you are not alone! You may not see them, but you would be surprised at the number of men who have discovered the sheer joy of spa treatments. It feels good, the phone doesn't ring, you can't be interrupted, and the relaxation is nothing short of heavenly. Women tend to know this sooner than men. For female physicians who are using spa relaxation as a necessary part of burnout recovery; they may find it becomes a lifetime habit!

Slow Action Items:

This list is adapted from the work of Dr. Herbert J. Dr.Freudenberger, (1926 – 1999), a German-born American psychologist. His most significant contribution to the field of medicine is the understanding and treatment of stress, burnout, and substance abuse. Freudenberger was one of the first to describe the symptoms of exhaustion professionally and to conduct a comprehensive study on burnout. In 1980, he published a book dealing with burnout, which became a standard reference on the syndrome. His most prestigious award was the American Psychological Foundation Gold Medal Award for Life Achievement in the Practice of Psychology, given to him in 1999.

Dr. Freudenberger drew up a profile of people who run a great risk of becoming burned out. According to Freudenberger they have the following qualities and habits:

- A perfectionist

- Conscientious

- Hard worker

- Dedicated and idealistic

- Ambitious

- Have the need to prove themselves

- Goal-oriented

- Find it difficult to say no

- Find it difficult to set boundaries

- Do more than they can

- Do more than they are asked to

- Unable to delegate

- Sacrifice themselves (their personal life) for the job

Many of these characteristics are what make us physicians. We are competitive and perfectionists so that we have what it takes to get into medical school. These traits help us tolerate and complete the rigors of the journey through residency, and enable us to excel in practice, caring for our patients for a very long time.

If you read through the list above several times, you may recognize that a few items are over-represented in your personality or character. This is important. Why? Because once you have identified these items you can make a mental list of what is "hurting" your ability to reach a balanced life. These traits are the ones you are going to concentrate on in your recovery from burnout syndrome. These could be considered your burnout "triggers" and you will have to learn to manage, even marginalize them, to get well and remain that way.

That said, right now, do nothing actionable about those traits. You have identified them, now we want you to sleep on it. Think about these things. Try to figure out when these characteristics first emerged- were you a young child, in high school, in college or in practice? These are important insights because eventually you will need to know which of these traits trigger burnout in order to develop effective strategies with which to manage them. Go back to the list in a few weeks, review it in light of your considerations and keep it close at hand.

Once you have completed the rapid action list, it is time to start working on making small incremental changes to these identified "trigger traits". The goal is to tone them down slightly and manage them in order to create more balance in your life. Realize that these "trigger traits" may be warriors in their own right. They will want to remain powerful and in control. They will want to win at all costs. You will have to be determined to recover from burnout in order to win these battles along the way but you can, and will.

Being a perfectionist

If you search the internet for "perfectionist" you will find that articles on burnout and stress are some of the first to appear on the list of results. Even the internet correlates the two! Being a perfectionist and being a physician creates enormous amounts of stress. You are in the business of treating human beings which are far from perfect, with science that although advanced is far from perfect, with imaging and drugs that can never be perfect. That is a recipe for crushing stress and burnout.

A study published in the journal Procedia - Social and Behavioral Sciences, called "Correlations between Perfectionism, Stress, Psychopathological Symptoms and Burnout in the Medical Field" substantiated the connection between the prevalence of perfectionism and burnout syndrome saying, "Our study indicated the fact that the associations between perfectionism tendencies, perceived stress, burnout and psychopathological symptoms in medical employees were positively and statistically significant. The burnout syndrome among the medical professionals negatively affects not only the individual and the organization, but also the patients. Most of the times, burnout represents a reaction to stress."

We all have been led to believe that being a perfectionist is a part of our personalities. Even if that is true, there are things you can do to give yourself a break from the punishing impact of being a perfectionist:

- Stop thinking in terms of giving 150%. Trying giving 80% once in a while and leave 20% to rejuvenate yourself.

- Practice congratulating yourself when a piece of a major project is completed successfully. Pace yourself and look at the small steps first. If when completed, the project is "near-perfect" you may be able to accept that, knowing that parts of it were absolutely perfect.

- Do you resist taking on new work for fear you won't be able to complete it perfectly? Set interim goals for yourself. Decide what factors will determine when each part of the project is completed and stick to your definition. Don't continually revisit and rework the work. This will prevent you from overreaching, and will allow you to pace yourself and mark your progress.

Conscientiousness is defined as a person wishing to do what is right, especially to do one's work or duty well and thoroughly. A conscientious person is described as being diligent, industrious, punctilious and painstaking.

Dr. John M. Oldham has defined the Conscientious personality style. The following eight characteristic traits and behaviors are listed in his The New Personality Self-Portrait.

- Hard work. The Conscientious person is dedicated to work, works very hard, and is capable of intense, single-minded effort.

- The right thing. To be Conscientious is to be a person of conscience. These are men and women of strong moral principles and values. Opinions and beliefs on any subject are rarely held lightly. Conscientious individuals want to do the right thing.

- The right way. Everything must be done "right," and the Conscientious person has a clear understanding of what that means, from the correct way to balance the checkbook, to the best strategy to achieve the boss's objectives, to how to fit every single dirty dish into the dishwasher.

- Perfectionism. The Conscientious person likes all tasks and projects to be complete to the final detail, without even minor flaws.

- Perseverance. They stick to their convictions and opinions. Opposition only serves to strengthen their dogged determination.

- Order and detail. Conscientious people like the appearance of orderliness and tidiness. They are good organizers, catalogers, and list makers. No detail is too small for Conscientious consideration.

- Prudence. Thrifty, careful, and cautious in all areas of their lives, Conscientious individuals do not give in to reckless abandon or wild excess.

- Accumulation. A "pack rat," the Conscientious person saves and collects things, reluctant to discard anything that has, formerly had, or someday may have value for him or her.

To further illustrate, Dr. Oldham lists high profile people as having a conscientious personality style, among them, Mohandas K. Gandhi, Al Gore, George Harrison, Thomas Jefferson, Sandra Day O'Connor, Michelle Obama, Yoko Ono, Ayn Rand, Carl Sagan, Jonathan Swift, Margaret Thatcher, George F. Will, Woodrow Wilson and many more.

Being conscientious is a good thing, so how does it contribute to burnout? Look at some of the words that Dr. Oldham uses to describe the personality type- intense, perfectionist, works very hard. These are some of the very same words used to describe burnout. Conscientious people hold within them many of the traits of burnout syndrome. Without careful management, it is easy to hit the slippery slope of burnout.

A study reported in the International Journal of Trade, Economics and Finance, called "How does Personality Affect Job Burnout?" confirmed this relationship. It concluded that "more conscientiousness leads to more burnout; maybe because high conscientiousness does not allow a person to be indifferent toward the job, so s/he is more exposed to job stress and burnout."

Yet, it seems a bit ridiculous to suggest that you become less conscientious. Instead, consider these tips to manage it so it doesn't lead to burnout:

- Take a break during the day. Get a cup of coffee or tea. You can be dedicated without working yourself into exhaustion.

- Learn to say no. You can say no to new projects if you are saturated. That doesn't mean you aren't conscientious, it means you are practicing time management.

- Ask for help. This isn't admitting defeat and it isn't slacking on the job. Asking for help, or creating a team or task force to work on a project is good work practice.

- Take time off. Working 7 days a week or never taking a vacation doesn't help anyone.

- You can be painstaking in attention to detail, without it becoming the adverse level of perfectionism that we discussed above. You can be conscientious in making sure you have followed through and paid attention to each detail of the work, without it leading to high anxiety and sleepless nights.

Working hard

Working hard is certainly a great ethic to have. We can see the difference in the lives of those who work hard and those who don't. However, Burnout syndrome blurs the line between working hard and working to avoid life's problems. Burying oneself in one's work to avoid thinking about life is not productive, it's dangerous. Working hard to meet some impossible, self-imposed bar of excellence will make you sick. Here is what you need to know- if you are driven to work hard because you want to achieve perfection, if your self-esteem is tied only to your achievements at work, it's time to take stock of exactly why you are working so hard.

Let's use a common analogy- "You can't see the forest for the trees."

Are you working so hard that you have forgotten the big picture?

Are you working to complete so many detailed tasks in your practice that you don't have time to grow it?

Have you lost the time to reenergize yourself so that you can be the compassionate doctor you set out to be?

Do you have your head down working in the office so much, that you have lost touch with the community? If you don't know what is going on, how can you effectively treat the citizens of the community?

Has your family given up asking you to do things because they now assume you will say you have too much work to go?

If you have answered yes to any of these questions, life may be passing you by. If you can no longer see the forest for the trees it may be time to look up and walk out of the forest for a while. A little sunshine will do you a lot of good.

A review of statistics and literature on the amount of work that Americans do each week shows that we work longer than people in other countries of the developed world. Whether or not we work harder is too subjective to measure. Online MBA says that in average, Americans work a 46 hour work week, while Denmark and Sweden have a 31 hour work week and Germany, Norway and the Netherlands have a 27 hour work week. Certainly you know people who work long hours because they want to, and they wear it like a badge of honor. Unfortunately, that is not going to work well for them in the long term. Online MBA reports that after 8 hours of work, productivity decreases by half, and increasing the work week from 40 to 60 hours, only yields an extra quarter of output. Other countries' workers are happier and healthier. We could learn from them.

Dedicated and idealistic

When thinking about the personal and professional cost of being selflessly dedicated and eternally idealistic, we came across this story by Dr. Karen Wyatt that was published in HuffPost Healthy Living. Dr. Wyatt is a hospice and family physician and the author of the award-winning book "What Really Matters: 7 Lessons for

Living from the Stories of the Dying." Her account of the price of being idealistic is gripping, and so we print it here as a warning of the dear price physicians pay for not being realistic in their practice.

"I remember so clearly all of the idealistic optimism I felt at the beginning of medical school: the naïve certainty that I was going to help people and save their lives... and I would do that through the power of love. Yes, I came to medicine with the awareness that love is actually the force that heals and I was determined to bring my knowledge of love to medical practice. It was going to be miraculous.

And I remember just as clearly the day when all of my idealism came crashing down around my feet, in my Waterloo moment, leaving me disillusioned and bereft. On that particular morning I was working in the emergency room as a fourth-year medical student when a trauma patient was brought in by ambulance.

She had been in an auto accident and had been ejected through the windshield because she wasn't wearing a seatbelt. We soon learned that she was just 16 years old and had been on her way to school, driving her best friend in the car she had received for her birthday just a few months before.

She had massive injuries to her head and neck, and the ER trauma team moved in quickly to begin resuscitation. I was assigned to help with chest compressions, monitor IV fluids and stay out of everyone else's way. In a blur of urgent yet efficient activity, dozens of people worked on the girl, performing their roles in this well-choreographed death-defying dance.

I helped wherever I was needed and watched and waited... for the miracle to occur. We were going to save her. This incredible super team of highly-skilled technicians with an endless supply of catheters, wires, tubes, syringes, plasma, and defibrillator paddles. She was only 16 -- just a few years younger than me. She would not die. We wouldn't let her go. I wouldn't let her go... I had love on my side after all. We just had to allow enough time for the miracle.

We worked on her for what seemed like an entire day, yet it may have been only an hour. One by one the technicians withdrew and left the little cubicle where the miracle was yet to take place. I stayed through everything, holding her hand, sending her all the love I could muster, believing... believing... she will not die.

But she did. The nurse removed all the tubing and wires and covered her lovely young face and curly blond, blood-caked hair with a clean sheet. We were giving up on the miracle. We were giving up on love.

I was devastated and broken apart -- all of this intense, focused effort had been for just one purpose: to save her life. And now, just like that, we were giving up. I stood there speechless trying to comprehend what had gone wrong -- did I not send enough love to her? Had I not believed strongly enough in the possibility of a miracle?

I wandered around the ER, trying to find someone to talk to about what had just happened, but the resident and attending were already working with other patients, the nurses were writing their notes and the orderlies were cleaning up, getting the cubicle ready for someone else. No one looked at me. No one noticed my pain. No one talked to me... ever... about the death of that girl, or about the death of any patient.

I went home that night and fell on my bed, exhausted and numb. When I tried to kick my shoes off I found that, for some reason, they were stuck on my feet and I had to struggle to remove them. Then I looked inside and saw that they were filled with dried blood -- the blood of the young girl had dripped down underneath the drape sheet while I held her hand, slowly filling my shoes without my awareness.

I crumpled onto the floor of my bedroom and sobbed and sobbed, holding onto those shoes that I would never wear again. I pictured the face of that beautiful girl, lying serenely on the gurney while her life slipped through our hands and her blood dripped into my shoes.

I understood in that moment for the first time the weight of the responsibility I was taking on my shoulders... on my heart... by becoming a doctor. The pain of losing that patient was overwhelming and the sorrow from the failed miracle was so immense it could drown me. I knew then that medicine would always be a life and death struggle... for the patient... and also for me. And I was no longer certain how it would turn out in the end. Miracles were suddenly hard to come by."

Ambitious

"Oh he will go far, he is so ambitious." "She has a great future ahead of her, she has been ambitious since the day she was born." How many times have you heard that?

Ambition is usually a character trait to be praised and admired. So why is it listed here as one of the traits that can lead to burnout? Because ambition uncontrolled, ambition "without borders" as it were, quickly becomes obsession.

Not to become a defacto dictionary, but one of the best ways to describe the two sides of the ambition coin is to talk about the meaning of the word. Ambitious is described as "eagerly desirous of achieving or obtaining success" and "an earnest desire for achievement or distinction". Those are all good things.

However, synonyms for ambitious begin to give us some insight into how ambition can go wrong; words like aggressive, anxious, driving, power-loving and zealous. Those words are not inclusive or collaborative. They are self-serving and narrow minded of purpose.

An ambitious person can also be described as someone who is competitive, demanding, difficult, pushy, and yes, even obsessed. One could argue that if an ambitious person did not have all of these traits, s/he would never achieve the success they so desire. That may be the case however they are also the traits that can lead to burnout. Competition does not allow you to rest or back down from a challenge. Being demanding does not lead you to discussion and the consideration of ideas; it can make you do nothing but deliver edicts. Being difficult does not gain you widespread support among your colleagues or staff. And all of these result in increased stress, longer work hours because you believe you are the only one who can "get it done right", and most likely sleepless nights.

The antonyms for ambitious include words like content, easy, fulfilled and satisfied. Look at the difference between the energy of those words and the ones listed above. These are calmer, softer, and filled with much less aggression.

We would argue that ambition is a good thing, if and when you understand it within a balanced view of your life. If you are naturally competitive, soften it with an easy manner. If you are obsessed with being chief of the department, ok go for it, but remember to be satisfied with your accomplishments along the way. Politics may not be on your side to give you that position, but you may be an extraordinary physician, and you need to make sure to give yourself that success. In fact, you may consider yourself a demanding boss, but when tempered with being satisfied when an employee does his or her best to meet your demands, you become a fair and balanced boss.

As with everything in life, ambition taken in reasonable amounts is a good thing. Ambition taken in large doses, to the exclusion of all other considerations will make you ill and hasten your slide into full-fledged burnout syndrome. It all comes down to how you define yourself as ambitious.

Having the need to prove yourself

Our egos can be nasty. If you have the need to prove yourself to others, it means that you don't believe in yourself in the first place. It means that you are operating from a position of self-doubt, and probably fear and uncertainty. If you need to prove yourself, then you feel that you have failed at something. You need to prove to others that you are a success, that their impression of you is wrong, that you are strong and skilled.

The problem with the need to prove yourself is that it is a race against an unknown clock. You are racing to always "show them" what you can do. You are running to catch up with a perception. It is an exhausting state of being.

One person, who will remain anonymous out of respect for his privacy, describes it like this: "Most of us as men are trying to prove things. We feel the need to prove ourselves smart, strong, right, desirable, sexy. We need to prove that we are loved. We feel the need to prove that we are capable. We try to prove that we are all-sufficient. We tend to use the people around us to prove these things. Ouch yet? If people laugh, we are funny and accepted. If our wives will do certain things for us, then she must really love us/desire us. If our kids don't obey us, then we must not be perfect… If people do what we demand of them, then we must be respectable/powerful. If our boss approves of us, then we must be competent and admired."

It's exhausting to read that. However, it provides a window into understanding how the need to prove oneself is a key ingredient for burnout syndrome.

The very fact that you may be heading toward burnout means that you will not take the time to reflect on why you feel you have to prove yourself to others, so we will assist you by listing some of the reasons here. See if any of these apply to you:

- You have to prove that your parents were wrong when they said you would never amount to anything.
- You have to prove your professor wrong- the one who said you didn't have what it takes to get through medical school.

- You have to prove the CEO wrong- the one who said you could never build a profitable practice.
- You have to prove your wife wrong, after all, she is the one who said you could never succeed enough to make helping you through medical school worthwhile.

What one thing do all of these have in common? They all occurred in the past, and yet, they keep you running today. These ghosts drive you to run faster, jump higher, and work longer to prove yourself.

The next question you need to ask yourself is "Who I am trying to prove myself to?" We know who it was in the past, but who are you trying to prove yourself to today? Do you really think they notice you are trying to prove yourself?

Marc Chernoff writes "practical tips for productive living" and he has some helpful thoughts on how to stop trying to prove yourself:

"Ignore the comparisons and expectations knocking at your door. The only person you should try to be better than is the person you were yesterday. Prove yourself to yourself, not others.

"Let go of the foolish need to prove yourself to everyone else, and you'll free yourself to accomplish what matters most to you. Sometimes you have to remind yourself that you don't have to always be and do what everyone else is being and doing.

"If you try too hard to impress everyone else with your "perfection," you will stunt your growth. You will spend all your time looking a certain way, instead of living a certain way."

Goal-oriented

Of course you are goal-oriented, would you be a physician today if you weren't? You have set goals for yourself for as long as you can remember. You probably started setting goals in elementary school, because that's what driven people do. If you are set on demonstrating your ability in "achievement situations", then you are considered a "goal- oriented person." Being goal oriented is a positive trait; it also one that can go sideways, and end up leading you on the path to burnout.

Moderation is the key. Brian Tracy is the author of "The Psychology of Achievement". In his personal success guidelines, he recommends being goal-oriented, but he also recommends being people and health oriented. In other words- being balanced. Here are some excerpts from his website on personal success:

"Be Goal Oriented. You need to be a habitual goal setter, and dedicate yourself to working from clear, written goals every day of your life. All highly successful people are intensely goal oriented. They know exactly what they want, they have it written down, they have written plans to accomplish it, and they both review and work on their plans every single day.

"Be People Oriented. This is where you put relationships in the center of your life. This is your decision to cultivate within yourself the habits of patience, kindness, compassion and understanding. Virtually all of your happiness in life will come from your ability to get along well with other people.

"Be Health Oriented. This means that you must fastidiously watch your diet, and always eat the right foods in the right proportions. You must exercise on a regular basis, continually using every muscle and joint of your body to keep it young and fit. And finally you must have good habits of rest and recreation that will enable you, in combination with diet and exercise, to live to be 80 or 90 years old. Remember, your health is the most important single thing you have, and it is completely subject to the habits that you develop with regard to the way you live."

So as you see, you can be "intensely goal oriented" without it taking over your life and becoming your sole reason for being in practice. When moderated with being people and health oriented, you can live intensely if you like, while avoiding burnout because you are in balance.

Finding it difficult to say no and finding it difficult to set boundaries

These are usually listed as two separate symptoms of burnout syndrome, however for the purposes of elaborating on them, they are so close as to be one. If you find it difficult to say no you have set no boundaries and if you have no boundaries then you will never say no.

Both men and women may have trouble saying no and setting boundaries, but the relationship-oriented biology of women sometimes leads them to suffer from this more frequently. In fact, the website Mommd, a resource that connects women in medicine, has dedicated quite a bit of space to this issue. This is what they have to say about setting boundaries;

"Boundaries are limits you set on how others can treat you or behave around you. People treat you as you allow them to; however, you can actually teach others how to treat you based on how strong or weak your boundaries are.

"Having strong boundaries are important for protecting your body, mind, and spirit. Setting boundaries can make an enormous impact on the quality of your life. It is a major step in taking control of your life and vital for taking responsibility for yourself and your life. It is the one skill that you most need to develop in order to create the kind of life you really want. However, it's often the area where most people seem to have the most difficulties.

"Setting strong boundaries will help you stand up for yourself, stop agreeing to do things you really don't want to do, and start feeling less guilty about putting your own needs first. It's a part of the process of defining yourself and what is acceptable to you. When you don't have boundaries set other people will step over the line without even realizing where it is.

"The first step in establishing boundaries is self-awareness; you'll need to identify where you need more space, self-respect, energy, and/or personal power. Begin this process by recognizing when you feel angry, frustrated, violated, or resentful. In these cases, you've often had a boundary "crossed". By becoming aware of situations that require you to have stronger limits, you can begin creating and communicating your new boundaries to others."

Remember, your goal is not to set rigid boundaries, but to set clear boundaries. Clear boundaries protect you and avoid misunderstanding because they are clearly communicated and consistently enforced.

Doing more than you can and more than you are asked to

Once again, these are two items that are listed as separate symptoms of burnout syndrome. However, they are so closely related that trying to elaborate on them separately would be redundant. Therefore, we will examine these two symptoms together.

Doing more than you can: Why would you do more than you can? Why would you take on more than you know you have the ability, time, or bandwidth to do? You may feel that doing more than you can will increase your visibility within the organization, it will position you as an expert or leader, or it is a way to prove yourself. In reality, the tendency to do more than you can is setting yourself up for failure.

By definition, "doing more than you can" means that your schedule is already full. Your time is blocked out with no room for additional commitments. You are already working long hours, and having trouble meeting family commitments. Now you are taking on more work, to prove to yourself and/or your colleagues that you can, except you can't. The end result will be that you make mistakes, deliver the product late, or fall down on completing it; the polar opposite of what you wanted to accomplish. If this is the result, why would you ever try to do more than you can?

In "Zen Habits" Leo Babauta writes about the philosophy of "simple productivity" which he calls Do Less. He says, "If you define "productivity" as a means of making the most of your actions, of the time you spend working (or doing anything), of being as effective as possible, then 'Do Less' is the best way to be productive.

"Consider: I can work all day in a flurry of frenetic activity, only to get a little done, especially when it comes to lasting achievement. Or I can do just a couple things that take an hour, but those are key actions that will lead to real achievement. In the second example, you did less, but the time you spent counted for more."

"Do less, but make every action count. Send fewer emails, but make them important. Write fewer words, but make each word essential. Really consider the impact of every action you take, and see if you can eliminate some actions. See if you can achieve a great impact doing less. This doesn't mean 'less is more'. It means 'less is better'."

The very thought of doing less may fly in the face of your work ethic and training. However, you are faced with burnout, a potentially life threatening, career ending syndrome that is not to be taken lightly. You must find some things to change in your life if you are to heal from burnout. Why not start with this philosophy? You can try it in one area of your work day and then build from there. In fact, as Leo suggests, try out this philosophy with your e-mails, and then slowly expand the new practice of Do Less into other areas of your work day.

Doing more than you are asked to

Parents often teach their children to always "do more than you are asked to" under the guise of teaching initiative. Business schools teach aspiring executives to always do more than they are asked to show that they are hungry for success and that they can think for themselves. However, a physician facing burnout should not be doing more than s/he is asked to do. Why? Because it is one more symptom of not having any boundaries, not being able to say no, feeding the need to prove oneself and all of the other traits that lead to the slippery slope of burnout syndrome.

This symptom, more than any of the others, may be difficult to understand as something that needs to be curtailed. After all, society is filled with admonitions to "do more than you think you can", "go the extra mile", and "stretch yourself".

For example:

Motivational Guru Gary Ryan Blair says "Do more than is required. What is the distance between someone who achieves their goals consistently and those who spend their lives and careers merely following? The extra mile."

General George Patton said, "Always do more than is required of you."

Lowell Thomas said "Do a little more each day than you think you can."

And Henry Drummond said "Unless a man undertakes more than he possibly can do, he will never do all that he can."

The prevalence of that philosophy makes it difficult to believe that doing more than you asked is actually a bad thing. However, there are two sides to the coin. Encouraging young people to work hard is good. Giving underachievers motivation is healthy. You are none of those. You are most likely a Type-A overachiever given to perfectionism and problem solving. You may also be headed for burnout. For you, the other side of the coin is more fitting.

For example:

Dr. Benjamin Spock said, "Trust yourself. You know more than you think you do."

Lucille Ball said, "I think knowing what you cannot do is more important than knowing

what you can."

And John Wooden said, "Just do the best you can. No one can do more than that."

For physicians struggling to make some sense of endless hours of work and an onslaught of changing government and insurance regulations, mergers, acquisitions, global coding changes, and increasingly conservative reimbursements, a change in work philosophy is in order.

Not being able to delegate

You can't delegate. You are not alone. Many managers find it difficult. If you are suffering from any stage of burnout, you will find delegation nearly impossible. Delegation requires trust and confidence in those to whom you delegate. It requires that you are able to let go of the task or the initiative at hand and entrust staff with responsibility. If you are burned out and have lost those relationships with staff, you are not going to be able to delegate.

Not being able to delegate can quickly become a patient care issue. Increasingly, hospitals are relying on care teams that involve physicians, nurses, therapists and support staff. Physicians must be able to work in this collaborative atmosphere and be willing to delegate patient care as appropriate to team members.

A study published in Health Policy Journal looked at delegation in a healthcare setting. The purpose of the study was to "explore the main facilitators and barriers to task reallocation" in healthcare settings. The impetus for the study was to find out if expanding the health care team would help to deal with any future shortage of physicians.

"One of the innovative approaches to dealing with the anticipated shortage of physicians is to reallocate tasks from the professional domain of medicine to the nursing domain. Various (cost-) effectiveness studies demonstrate that nurse practitioners can deliver as high quality care as physicians and can achieve as good outcomes. However, these studies do not examine what factors may facilitate or hinder such task reallocation."

Highlights of the study show that there is work to be done to accomplish widespread physician acceptance of delegating patient care to other clinicians. The study "systematically reviewed task reallocation from cure (physicians) to care (Nurse Practitioners)" and found four categories of facilitators and barriers. The study found that addressing those facilitators and barriers to task reallocation is a dynamic process, and that "task reallocation to NPs requires reframing of professional boundaries. Researchers concluded that "Professionalism should be reframed at the multiple layers of the healthcare system. Introducing nurse practitioners in healthcare requires organizational redesign and the reframing of professional boundaries. Especially the facilitators and barriers in the analytical themes of 'professional boundaries' and 'organizational environment' should be considered when reallocating tasks. If not, these factors might hamper the cost-effectiveness of task reallocation in practice."

In simple terms, physicians find it difficult to delegate, even to accomplished colleagues. There is a lesson in that for physicians struggling with the symptoms of burnout. One might suggest that the forward thinking segments of the health care system are trying to expand care teams, both to increase patient safety and reduce pressure on available physicians. Participating in those teams, and finding a way to delegate might create healthier physicians with career longevity and less burnout.

Sacrificing yourself

Martyrs went the way of the Diocletian era in the 4th century, and yet physicians experiencing burnout syndrome believe that sacrificing themselves to the practice of medicine is a lofty goal. They feel that they must sacrifice themselves in order to effectively run the practice, care for patients, fulfill on call hours and make a profit. What it really means is that the physician is out of balance and has lost perspective.

If you feel this way, you should take stock of the root cause. Do you feel you must sacrifice yourself because you are the only one who can do the work? Are you depressed and feel as though there is nothing else to do but use yourself up for the good of your patients?

A couple of years ago the locum tenens staffing firm Weatherby Healthcare conducted a survey that found, not surprisingly, that physicians were not practicing what they preached to their patients regarding a healthy lifestyle. We venture a guess that these statistics have not changed; if anything they are probably worse now:

- 82 percent of those surveyed forgo personal activities such as hobbies, working out, and family time because of busy work schedules.
- 44 percent of physicians say they don't have time to exercise because of busy work schedules.

- 43 percent don't go on vacations
- 42 percent forgo their hobbies
- 41 percent would like more time for volunteer work
- 38 percent miss out on family time

Many physicians feel they must retire, close their practice, or even change careers to achieve a work-life balance and avoid burnout.

Medical schools and healthcare institutions have traditionally considered self-sacrifice and self-denial the cornerstones of a physician's life. It is generally accepted, beginning in medical school that physicians should learn to ignore their own well-being. This self-denial actually leads to a lower quality of patient care. As physicians experience increased stress and depression, their ability to think clearly and make exacting care decisions becomes clouded. They may order too many tests to protect themselves, exposing the patient to undue procedures and increasing the cost of healthcare. Exhaustion begins to deplete the physician's ability to develop productive, healing relationships with patients. In the worst case scenario, self-sacrifice and the other harmful symptoms of burnout lead to physician suicide, which occurs at six times the rate of the general population.

The importance of physician wellness is put under a bright light in a study published in the Journal of Family Medicine that was conducted at Duke University. The study found that when coaching was made available to physicians, and helped them along the path to self-care, patient care improved as well.

"This study suggests that physician well-being coaching can help raise participant self-awareness, increase the value placed on self-care and allow for new perspectives and approaches for increasing well-being. Physicians reported that coaching positively influenced the way they related to their patients and brought about greater compassion and empathy.

"Health and well-being coaching interventions for patients are increasingly integrated into clinics and hospitals throughout the U.S. They offer patients a valuable bridge between self-care and healthcare. Despite marked increases in demands and pressures on

physicians, similar interventions are rarely offered to them. Making such interventions more accessible for physicians requires working upstream, but the benefits of healthier health providers can pay dividends for generations to come. Cultivating a culture of self-care and compassion in medicine is a vital place to start."

Resources and references:

Procedia - Social and Behavioral Sciences

Volume 127, 22 April 2014, Pages 529–533

The International Conference PSYCHOLOGY AND THE REALITIES OF THE
CONTEMPORARY WORLD – 4th EDITION - PSIWORLD 2013
http://www.sciencedirect.com/science/article/pii/S1877042814023957

International Journal of Trade, Economics and Finance, Vol. 2, No. 2, April 2011

How does Personality Affect on Job Burnout? Mohammad Reza Akhavan Anvari, Nader Seyed
Kalali, and Aryan Gholipour

http://www.ptypes.com/conscientious.html

http://www.prdaily.com/Main/Articles/Most_employed_Americans_work_more_than_40_hours_pe
_12123.aspx

http://www.pickthebrain.com/blog/why-hard-work-isnt-such-a-good-idea/

http://www.huffingtonpost.com/healthy-living/

Karen M. Wyatt, M.D. Become a fan

Author, 'What Really Matters: 7 Lessons for Living from the Stories of the Dying'

When Doctors Grieve

Posted: 03/06/2015 11:37 am EST Updated: 03/06/2015 11:59 am EST

http://touchingyourcommunity.com/tag/need-to-prove-oneself/ post by Chris Legg, 11/6/14 http://www.marcandangel.com/2013/11/24/7-reasons-to-stop-proving-yourself-to-everyone-else/

Marc and Angel Hack Life- Practical Tips for Productive Living

7 Reasons to Stop Proving Yourself to Everyone Else, written by, Marc Chernoff

http://en.wikipedia.org/wiki/Goal_orientation

http://www.mommd.com/settingboundaries.shtml, Copyright 2003 by Natalie Gahrmann

http://zenhabits.net/the-lazy-manifesto-do-less-then-do-even-less/

Reframing professional boundaries in healthcare: A systematic review of facilitators and barriers to task reallocation from the domain of medicine to the nursing domain

Maartje G.H. Niezencorrespondenceemail, Jolanda J.P. Mathijssenemail

Tilburg University, Department Tranzo, Netherlands

Open AccessArticle has an altmetric score of 4

DOI: http://dx.doi.org/10.1016/j.healthpol.2014.04.016

showArticle Info

http://www.healthpolicyjrnl.com/article/S0168-8510(14)00115-8/abstract

12 THE BIG PICTURE

A road map is the best way to approach dealing with burnout syndrome. This road map reflects our understanding of the problem and its origins, the literature, and the political atmosphere. It may contradict many of the prevalent explanations; it may be harsh to hear for some who are entrenched in their corporate/organization's belief system, especially those who have only worked in one organization throughout most of their career.

 In other words, for the most part, this chapter reflects our due diligence in researching the problem, our opinion and thoughts about the syndrome.

This is a non-scientific approach, and some may perceive it as a piece of fiction about health care. We say yes to all, as long as it will help you organize your thoughts into a road map for self-discovery, and a self-help tool regarding burnout.

This is in no way meant to be a call for action, but we hope it will inspire physician leaders to become interested in writing, in much more scientific method beyond the limits of this publication, about the items in this chapter. We also hope they will earnestly pursue more in-depth, articulate solutions to the difficult problems that lead to burnout syndrome.

There will be content addressing some of these issues, while some other issues are left for your imagination and own mental debate.

The road map is divided into the following categories:

1- Issues physicians cannot do something about.
2- Issues physicians can do something about as a group.
3- Issues physicians can do something about as individuals.

<u>Issues physicians cannot do something about</u>

I- Issues that serve as valves to control patient access to physician services:

We are not blind to the value and strong arguments behind each of these issues in optimizing patient care, outcomes, or saving dollars by the proposed mechanism for a particular intervention.

But we have developed the sense, right or wrong, while researching the subject that these valves are very practical in generating $ (x) % savings of health care cost, independent of their well justified reasoning. This is achieved by the mere fact that they can decrease patient access to care on a short term basis and accomplish the savings very effectively.

It is best for experienced economists to calculate how much (x) represents in dollars. But for the sake of argument let us give it a value of 0.5%,

knowing that the USA cost of health in 2012 was 3 trillion dollars. The x then, represents $ 3,000,000,000,000. 0.5% savings using these "valves" will produce savings of $15,000,000,000. Imagine, this $15 billion dollars a year was saved simply by limiting patient access to care.

To help you relate this number to something tangible, we copied the following paragraph from the Mayo Clinic website:

"Mayo Clinic reported annual revenue of $8.8 billion for 2012. Mayo, a not-for-profit, has more than 61,000 employees and treats more than 1 million patients each year from roughly 135 countries. As part of our operational plan in 2012, Mayo Clinic expected expenses to grow faster than revenue; expenses rose 9.6 percent, to $8.4 billion."

This is a list of the most important "valves" we could identify:

1- Small increments of declining payments by third party payers
2- Increasing documentation burdens
3- Increasing regulatory burdens
4- Increasing imposed financial punishments for not meeting evidence- based criteria of best practices

Before you reject any of these as patient access control valves, consider that any of these interventions used skillfully can lead to a decrease in the ability of physicians to see patients. The physician pool is limited, hence payments for health care expenses is limited by the ability of patients to see a physician.

II- Issues that are key to political elections. There is a good understanding among all political parties of the bottom line as it relates to these issues, but there is significant political difficulty in presenting a global solution. Rather, political parties are in the practice of offering micro-solutions that are inflated into macro-solutions during election cycles. In medical terms, it is very much like prescribing acetaminophen for the early stages of sepsis. You all know that the best outcomes can actually be achieved in this stage by identifying the pathogen and starting appropriate IV antibiotics. Anything short of that will result in circulatory collapse when compensatory mechanisms and homeostasis fail.

III- Government

Even with lobbying, interest groups, and political shifts, the United States government will act in the national interest only when health care issues become a national crisis. An aging population, new medical inventions, and shrinking Medicare funds are moving the issue quickly toward a national crisis. It is possible that we will arrive at that crisis stage in the first half of the 21 century.

Most of us have a rough idea of what a national crisis solution for health care would be.

IV- The need to become big

Entities like Kaiser-Permanente, Dignity health and many others can thrive only by getting bigger. Indeed, they do not have a choice. These entities can only grow as big as a "Nationalized Health System". In other words, as they grow bigger, the boundaries which differentiate them from what a national health system will look like are going to be so vague that it will be hard to tell the difference.

V- Giving up practice autonomy in exchange for financial security. We have discussed this topic in more detail in another chapter. We admit that some physicians have succeeded in tilting the equation in favor of practice autonomy; and as a by-product they have improved quality of care and patient satisfaction. This new breed of physicians is the concierge medicine practice. However, the following factors render it an ineffective method to deliver care to the United States population on a national level.

These issues are:

1- The concierge model may be applicable in primary care; it is not very applicable in specialty care.

2- The entrepreneurial risk tolerance needed for such a practice model is high, something very few physicians are comfortable taking on.

3- The percent of concierge physicians is very small when compared to the total physician work force. Contrary to what many others speculate will be overwhelming growth in the future, we do not think this is going to happen. We speculate that there will be a constellation of small caliber "concierge services" in many of the independent primary care practices. A version of this is offered already by "One Medical Group" an innovative medical group that was started in San Francisco and has significant, but modest penetration, into other metropolitan areas. In short, the concierge model works whereby a modest, reasonable monthly or yearly fee is paid by patients to the practice, in exchange for more prompt access to physician appointments, as well as better e-mail communication between patients and physicians, and sometimes house visits.

Issues physicians can do something about as a group

Do not expect to hear that unionizing, lobbying, or organizing formally is what we are going to discuss here. This stems from the fact that in our estimation the current problematic equation is simple: there are limited funds and growing expenses for physician practices. What we are suggesting here is that physicians as a group take on strategic planning in order to better prepare their work force for the changes that are coming. Also, we would suggest that physicians learn from their colleagues in Great Britain about the long term outcomes of such strategic planning. These suggestions are:

I-   Develop an infra-structure of physician managers. This has begun to occur on a smaller scale by physicians pursuing management degrees like MBAs; and on a larger scale in medical groups like Kaiser-Permanente. This is not enough. A small army of skilled physician managers is essential for the future if we are to successfully battle burnout. Supportive management is one of the key elements in overcoming burnout syndrome.

II-   Decrease expectations of what the real income is for working full time. Currently the gross income for physicians reflects working at a capacity of 120-130% rather than 100%. Kaiser-Permanente, again, has invented a smart remedy to solve this problem. Physicians are allowed to decrease their work load when calculating time from 100% as a full time, down to 70-90% as part-time. The organization maintains the full scope of benefits for the physician, such as health insurance, retirement, and partnership opportunities. These are not affected by becoming a part-time physician. This innovative approach helps many physicians attend to family needs, have children, or just decrease their work load when unable to work full-time for personal reasons.

However, we think that this option is frequently utilized by many full-time physicians who are trying to manage their burnout. Those physicians decrease their work load for few years until they find a balance in their life, then they go back to working full-time. We do not have access to the percent of physicians who elect not to go back to being full-time and instead choose to remain working at 80% or 90% of full-time. We think that a simple survey of the physicians who utilize this amazing benefit, as well as ones who do not return to 100% full-time, would be fascinating. The opportunity to ask them why they chose a certain level of work hours would give us a rough idea about the burnout status of physicians in a well-managed organization like Kaiser-Permanente. The entire health care system would be learn so much from such a survey/study.

III-   Develop national counseling groups for physician spouses to help them become an effective tool in protecting physicians from developing burnout. It has been a consistent research finding that having a supportive spouse or partner is a protective variable against physician burn out. The best qualified organizations to spearhead such an effort are the state medical associations. They can understand the state market place better than other entities and fine tune their programs to accommodate local needs.

IV-   Develop physician-oriented courses to educate them about the signs, symptoms, and management of burnout. This task is best carried by the specialty academies like the American College of Physicians, American Academy of Family Practice and so on. The American Medial Association can contribute tremendously to developing these courses at a national level.

V-   Develop non-physician manager courses to help them better understand the dynamics of physicians as a group. The bottom line is to help managers convert their thinking from managing physicians as a commodity, to handling them more effectively and productively as assets.

VI-   Invest in developing better Electronic Medical Records (EMR) that serve patient-physician interaction, rather than its current role of a sophisticated tracking system of activity. For the most part, EMR has only added more non-medical work to physicians' schedules. These changes are best accomplished by the Federal Government that could appropriate substantial research funds directly to academic teaching and research institutions like MIT and Stanford. These funds would facilitate the R&D necessary to develop useful technology to improve EMR. Currently EMR is nothing more than a fancy "spread sheet" that uses a sizable portion of physicians' medical time and essentially turns them into low-paid data entry personnel. The return on this investment as a nation could be tremendous.

Issues physicians can do something about as individuals

We are going to discuss these action items by dividing them into two categories. One category contains easy interventions that physicians can use to combat burnout. The second category lists difficult interventions to combat burnout.

Easy interventions:

1- Read this self-help book in its entirety. It is a good place to start to initiate self-guided debate about the extent of burnout in your day-to-day life.

2- Encourage the physician's spouse or partner to read the entire book as well.

3- Use this book as a trigger for relationship discussions with different groups: personal friends and family members, colleagues, managers, and support staff. Discussions can be approached differently with each of these groups.

4- Seek professional help from a trained psychologist. The main purpose of this is to learn about and validate the different feelings that physicians may experience in any given stage of Burnout syndrome.

5- Meet with colleagues in the work place once a month to discuss "frustrations" induced by the work environment

6- Take on a new hobby.

Difficult interventions:

1- Involve spouses or partners in learning how to be a better ingredient of the physician support system.

2- Share a positive contribution made in the physician's medical practice, with a spouse or partner on a weekly basis. There should be specific time set aside for this, possibly called "I made a difference in someone's life this week".

3- Bring the romance back into the relationship.

4- Spend more time with family and friends.

5- Decrease the work load.

6- Downgrade what is considered as acceptable gross income for your specialty.

7- Conduct an in-depth search to find more value in practicing medicine.

8- Devote time to doing something meaningless and fun. For example, Google "Lady Gaga" to laugh at her outrageous costumes and don't feel guilty about using the time! Do not consider it wasted time. Any "guilty pleasure" is easy to find as most of them appear on the front pages of any media source.

9- Spend more time with a limited number of patients every week to raise the appointments to the level of a self-gratifying visit. This time is best invested in visits where the patient does not have a very complex history. The goal is not to make a rare diagnosis. The goal is to accomplish spending time with a patient so that the visit meets falls into the category of "why physicians go into medicine in the first place". Having such visits will help to anchor physicians, and involve them in a process that reminds them of the value in practicing medicine.

This is free time offered by the physician. on top of all the free time physicians are forced to contribute to their patients. This will sound contradictory at first glance, but indeed it is an "investment" in their career in the form of "free time". This is completely different from the "free time" they are forced to contribute when pressured by third party payers, government regulations, and management.

10- Maintain self-care through nutrition and exercise.

11- Adapt a healthy philosophical outlook on the work.

12- Have a good mentor early on, and solid administrative support later in the career cycle.

13- Take vacation and travel time.

14- Set self-limits.

To elaborate on this subject more, we tap into a published study assessing the strategies that the annual winners of the American Medical Association "Foundation's Pride in the Profession Award" implement to fight burnout. Those well-adjusted physicians implement "Setting limits" as the first intervention:

These physician set limits through self-regulation by adhering to the following items:

Recognizing their body signaling them "Tension scale is going up", Examples:

Starting to get tense shoulders and neck

Stopping at the gas station to get a chocolate bar

Gaining a few extra pounds

What is next?

They act on these cues by applying their own healing remedies:

Realizing that you cannot do everything for everybody

Reaching out for support

Trying not to compromise with the philosophy: "When I am away, I am away.

Having a realistic goal, by subscribing to this statement: "I did the best I could under the circumstances."

Decreasing the work load

As we discussed earlier, these physicians regularly spend time with family and friends. Please note: they avoid counting travel for a conference as family time.

They maintain self-care through exercise.

They avoid listening to educational material during their exercise and/or work out; this is the time to rejuvenate.

Also, consider actively playing with pets as a healing exercise, even though it may not meet formal criteria for aerobic exercise.

These well-adjusted physicians also maintain self-care through relaxation:

- Taking take time off to listen to music
- Knitting
- A few extra hours of sleep
- Playing music

- Meditation
- Visiting a farmer's market
- Wandering through eclectic shops
- Hiking trips
- Being outdoors in nature has a very powerful restorative healing effect, use it to your advantage.

Relaxation is a time for healing with no goals or small achievements set as a secondary gain. There should be no concomitant tasks to boost the utilization of the time you have set aside for relaxation and self-healing.

In short, IT IS OK TO SET TIME FOR DOING NOTHING......... RELAX

Indeed our iPhone application "Relax-Templeton Neurology" is the perfect example for addressing what we as physicians call "wasting time". It is an excellent tool to bring down your pulse rate, and steel you from your current stress. It is free and to obtain the maximum benefit we recommend using it with an ear piece. Sit in a darkened room, and be patient. Your session should last a minimum of 5 minutes.

Enough with the promotion let us get back to the study.

Another thing those self-healing physicians applied was:

Humor:

The healing power of humor is incredibly powerful, either by being the comedian yourself and cracking jokes, or being the listener laughing at comedy as part of the audience. Overall it is essential to make an effort to maintain a sense of humor; it helps tremendously to maintain sanity in this health care atmosphere.

Self-healing physicians also:

Develop the skill to maintain balance in life. Meditation, exercise, relaxation, and vacations, when implemented separately and rarely, are not sufficient to maintain a balance in life. These activities should be components of an "all over plan" that is regularly and consistently implemented to achieve a balanced life. Aspirin will relieve the pain of an injured muscle, but it is not the appropriate approach to manage muscle injury and pain if it is caused by poorly fitting running shoes.

The well-adjusted, self-healing physicians that we have been talking about are also very good at putting things into prospective. They understand that physicians identify caring for others as their primary objective, yet they realize the need to include self-compassion in their careers.

Again, we inject our own opinion here: A physician's work and life is a living organism, it is an organic existence and cannot be separated into silos completely. As much as we try to shield our loved ones from the daily suffering we deal with, we physicians may need to bring our loved ones into our daily experience so that they can appreciate the good that we bring into peoples' lives.

ABOUT THE AUTHOR

AMR AL-HARIRI, MD

I Invest in Positive, Let it Flow into Your Life

A practicing Neurologist in California with the following certifications:

American Board of Psychiatry and Neurology

American Board of Internal Medicine

American Board of Pediatrics

This book is the first in a series about improving outcomes in medicine. This is not a simple formula that can be followed, it is a continuous implementation process of positive attributes.

What do you call the situation of a physician that accept insurance or Medicare, employed or an independent contractor, and feels that reimbursement continues to decline unfairly, while unable to take action to change the situation?

I call it a "job misfit", this is the seed that carries the risk of evolving into a burn out syndrome.

This comprehensive book is a must investment in the career of physicians, and their families; it is likely to pay dividends for years to come in a much better quality of life and productivity.

This is a must read for physicians' spouses and partners. You may have thought you knew the physician you sleep next to very well. But we assure you, you did not!

If you are a CEO or executive, health care consultant, a manager in a health care facility or organization, a health insurance strategist, or a politician; and you have the gut feeling that the tools available for you to thrive are not working out... I can help you serve your clients (the patients) to the level that your conscious dictate. The first step is to understand the problem. This is what this book is about

Once you have the problem dissected it is your nature and skill to develop your own, situation unique, strategies to maximize your return on investment in your most valuable assets: The Physicians; not the hospital building or the state of the art MRI.

"The Healthcare CEO" series addresses your needs

You are sophisticated, educated, capable and dedicated; this is why you are the CEO, the manager, the executive or consultant.

This is why this series is so different, but the right one for you.

I present you with a collection of building blocks; each of them is a unique concept by itself. Each one of them can be plugged into your organization independently and make a difference. Yet you can build an amazing structure from the ground up using all these building blocks.

It is you, the CEO, the chief engineer of your company's culture structure that can decide which blocks, when, and how.